Shared Care for
Prostatic Diseases

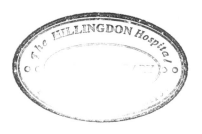

Shared Care for
Prostatic Diseases

Second Edition

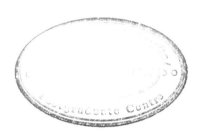

by
Roger Kirby MA MD FRCS (Urol) FEBU
Consultant Urologist, St George's Hospital, London, UK

John Fitzpatrick MCh FRCSI FRCS FEBU
Professor of Surgery, University College, Dublin, Ireland

Michael Kirby MB BS LRCP MRCS MRCP
Family Practitioner, The Surgery, Nevells Road, Letchworth, UK
and Director, Hertnet, Hertfordshire Primary Care Network,
UK

Andrew Fitzpatrick MB BCh MRCGP DCH DObst (RCPI)
Family Practitioner, Peel View Medical Centre, Kirkintilloch,
Glasgow, UK

I S I S
MEDICAL
M E D I A

© 2000 by Isis Medical Media Ltd.
59 St Aldates
Oxford OX1 1ST, UK

First published 2000

British Library Cataloguing-in-Publication Data.
A catalogue record for this title is available
from the British Library.

ISBN 1 901865 60 6

Kirby, R. (Roger)
Shared Care for Prostatic Diseases
Roger Kirby, John Fitzpatrick, Michael Kirby, Andrew Fitzpatrick (eds)

Always refer to the manufacturer's Prescribing
Information before prescribing drugs cited in this book.

Medical artwork by
Dee McLean

Design, illustrations and typesetting by
In Perspective Ltd.

Repro by
Track Direct, Middlesex, UK

Isis Medical Media staff
Commissioning Editor: John Harrison
Editorial Controllers: Sarah Carlson, Fiona Cornell
Production Manager: Sarah Sodhi

Printed and bound through
Phoenix Offset, Hong Kong
Printed in China

Distributed in the USA by
Books International, Inc., P.O. Box 605,
Herndon, VA 20172, USA

Distributed in the rest of the world by
Plymbridge Distributors Ltd., Estover Road,
Plymouth PL6 7PY, UK

Contents

Preface

It is now 7 years since we wrote the first edition of *Shared Care for Prostatic Diseases* and so much has happened since then that we felt a second edition was required. When we originally conceived the concept of the *Shared Care* series there was some scepticism expressed concerning the willingness of family practitioners to become involved in what was seen as a surgical disease area. The interim period has seen a surge in the use of medical therapy for benign prostatic hyperplasia (BPH), and unparalleled public and media interest in prostate cancer. As a consequence, the family physician is now dealing with more and more patients with prostatic disease, and it has become clear that referrals, each and everyone of them, for a specialist opinion is simply not feasible. Instead, the informed and educated family doctor will wish to examine and evaluate his patients, referring on those who require specialist appraisal by a urologist and initiating appropriate medical therapy for the straight forward case of uncomplicated BPH.

With this in mind, we have extensively updated this book, providing more evidence based information about BPH, prostate cancer and prostatitis, together with clear guidelines on who should or should not be referred. We have also provided up-to-date information about the latest advances in medical, and surgery therapy of these diseases. We hope that the book will be of value for those involved in the care of the very many men who suffer quality of life impairment as a result of prostatic disease.

Roger Kirby
John Fitzpatrick
Michael Kirby
Andrew Fitzpatrick

Foreword

When the first edition of *Shared Care for Prostatic Diseases* was published there was a degree of paranoia expressed by the urologists and trepidation expressed by the generalists. Care of patients with prostatic disease at that time was clearly in the domain of the urologist. However, as time has passed, the concept of shared care for patients with various diseases has now become the norm not the exception. Especially in the United States, when managed care is mandated, there is an expansion of duties for the primary care physician (PCP) with restricted referral to the specialist. Thus, the PCP has taken on more responsibility. With responsibility comes the need for education. This book is exactly the prescription for the education of the PCP with carefully screened information distilled by two internationally known urologists.

In the first chapter the authors give the rationale for shared care of men with prostatic disease. It is clear that with a limited workforce of urologists around the world, coupled with a more aware population and increased longevity, it is beyond the capability of the urologic community to care totally for men with prostatic disease. Moreover, epidemiological studies have revealed that there are a significant number of men who, up until recently, simply have not admitted that they had symptoms due to prostatic disease for fear of surgical intervention. The authors carefully outline the array of alternative therapies, both medical and minimally invasive, that have been added to the armamentarium of the PCP and urologist for the care of these patients. Thus, with more public awareness of both benign prostatic hyperplasia and prostate cancer, this book, amongst a number of books directed towards the public, can be expected to result in more men coming to their PCP inquiring as to the appropriate treatment of their specific problem. Indeed, this book ends with a series of very realistic case studies as well as oft-answered questions as a guide to the PCP.

If there is any fault to the book, it is simply the limitation of what is known. Thus, alternative therapies for localized prostate cancer are given with the caveat that prospective randomized trials have never been done. The choice of radiation versus surgery is a joint decision made by the treating physician with the patient and his family. Similarly, the authors are handicapped by the fact that new intermediate therapies directed against benign prostatic hyperplasia often are not subjected to rigorous randomized control trials and the efficacy of some of the techniques appear to be more in the eye of the initial investigator and company sponsoring the techniques than subsequent clinical experience demonstrates.

However, despite these limitations, the authors discuss in a clear fashion all of the current alternative treatments for patients with these diseases. They also include a segment involving the difficult topic of prostatitis or pelvic pain syndrome in the male.

The first edition of this book successfully accomplished its task. This edition includes modifications of old treatments and the addition of new modalities, bringing it into the new millennium. The book is valuable to the PCP as they address an ever-increasing number of patients with these diseases and ever-increasing array of different choices of treatment.

E Darracott Vaughan Jr MD Chairman
Department of Urology
Weill Medical College of Cornell University
New York-Presbyterian Hospital
New York, USA

The shared care concept

Shared care for prostatic disease involves the joint management of men with prostate problems by family practitioners and urologists. Like many new ideas, this concept was born out of necessity to manage change constructively. Traditionally, the diagnosis and management of prostatic disorders was handled exclusively by urologists for whom there was usually a relatively simple decision – to operate or not to operate. Two developments, in particular, have combined to challenge this *modus operandi*:

- Epidemiological surveys suggest that mild-to-moderate symptoms of benign prostatic hyperplasia (BPH) are extremely prevalent in men who do not seek the advice of either their family practitioner or a urologist [1].
- The availability of new treatment options for BPH have made men reluctant to accept transurethral resection of the prostate (TURP) as first-line therapy, favouring medical and other less invasive alternatives instead.

QUALITY OF LIFE

Disorders of the prostate are a major source of discomfort and disease in middle-aged and elderly men. Almost half of all men over the age of 65 years suffer some symptoms of bladder outflow obstruction caused by BPH [1,2], which often significantly reduce their quality of life [3–5].

Furthermore, prostate cancer is now the second most common cause of cancer death in men in many countries.

Over the coming years, family practitioners and urologists alike will see a steady increase in the number of patients who present with prostate problems. One important reason for this is the increase in life expectancy which has resulted in a continuing rise in the proportion of the world's population over 60 years of age (Fig. 1.1) [6]. Another reason is the increasing public awareness that the bothersome symptoms of BPH can now be treated with either new medical therapies or minimally invasive, short-stay surgery rather than procedures that require hospital admission and anaesthetic. Based on recent epidemiological data, in Europe, for example, to submit all those men over the age of 60 years whose quality of life is negatively affected by the symptoms of BPH to surgery would entail increasing the current TURP rate more than 10-fold and dramatically increasing the number of fully trained urologists [4].

Attitudes toward prostate cancer are also changing. Men in their so-called 'third age' (50–75 years) no longer consider themselves old, and are less prepared to accept that a reduced quality of life, because

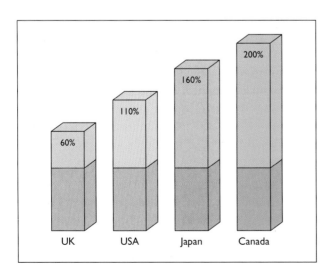

Figure 1.1. Projected percentage increase in population over 60 years of age by the year 2020. As the world's population ages, a steady increase in the number of patients who present with prostate problems is expected.

of waning health, is an inevitable accompaniment to the passage of time. Men's health is now firmly on the agenda [7]. Earlier diagnosis and improved methods of treatment are also commonly featured in the media, and men are increasingly pressing their doctors for a 'prostate health check'. Prostate disease will therefore have an increasing impact on health economics [8], which raises the question – how can these patients best be managed and who should look after them?

SHARED CARE – MEETING THE NEED FOR TREATMENT

The challenge, therefore, is to evolve a strategy that permits rapid access to diagnosis and treatment by urologists for those patients with the most need of more specialist evaluation and intervention (e.g. men under 75 years with significant volume prostate cancer or those with severely obstructive or complicated BPH). By contrast, those with only minor symptoms or moderate and no evidence of coexistent prostate cancer, who were formerly candidates for 'watchful waiting' in urology clinics, can be appropriately cared for by well informed and appropriately educated family practitioners. This process has been termed 'shared care'.

Advantages of a shared-care approach

The overall benefit of shared care for prostatic disease is improved patient care. However, its advantages to all those involved can be significant (Table 1.1). Indeed, far from reducing the diagnosis of prostate cancer, the wider introduction of shared care and medical therapy should increase the detection of early potentially curable lesions. Furthermore, in these times of increasing budgetary restrictions in most healthcare systems, a shared-care approach is likely to be more cost-effective than other approaches and therefore to be encouraged internationally by the governments and insurance companies who hold the purse-strings. Shared care implies a partnership between urologists, family practitioners and patients.

Table 1.1 Advantages of a shared-care approach for prostatic diseases

Patients
Reduced hospital visits and waiting times
Easier access to local medical advice
Greater continuity of treatment and better follow-up
Greater contact with the family practitioner, who is more aware of the
patient's medical and social history

Family practitioners
Patients may be more open with healthcare professionals with whom
they are familiar
Opportunity for family practitioners to broaden their knowledge of
prostatic disease and develop new skills
Rewards of team working and providing better patient care

Urologists
Reduced hospital admissions and surgical waiting times
Encourages more appropriate referrals
Earlier diagnosis of prostate cancer
More time available for patients who require specialist management
Rewards of stronger relations with community physicians and providing
better patient care

Raising awareness

The key to advancing this concept of shared care is to raise awareness of the prevalence and importance of both BPH and prostate
cancer, not only among the general public, but also among family
practitioners. Population-based surveys have shown a generally low
level of public knowledge relating to the prostate although this is
now changing. In addition, family practitioners sometimes seem
bewildered by the diseases that afflict this organ: a survey of family
practitioners in London, UK, revealed that the majority performed
less than five digital rectal examinations (DREs) a month [9]. This

strongly suggests that middle-aged and elderly men whose quality of life is being affected adversely by prostatic disease ascribe the symptoms to ageing, and do not trouble their family practitioner. Furthermore, the prostate seldom attracts specific enquiry in most standard health checks. The result – problems remain neglected, underdiagnosed and untreated.

Prostate disease – the three questions

In fact, the first step in detecting prostate disease, which is very simple for a family practitioner to undertake at a routine visit, is to ask the so-called 'three questions':

- Do you get up at night to pass urine?
- Is your urinary stream reduced?
- Are you bothered by bladder symptoms ('your waterworks')?

Most afflicted patients will give an affirmative to at least two of the three questions, and then the severity of the problem can be quantified by asking the patient to complete an International Prostate Symptom Score (IPSS) sheet (see pages 62–63).

THE LOGISTICS OF SHARED CARE

As family practitioners have become more conversant with the management of the specific disease processes, such as diabetes, asthma, hypertension and lipid disorders, they have become increasingly expert in selecting those cases most appropriate for specialist referral. This process has been supported by educational back-up from the specialists involved. Similar support will also be necessary when considering the logistics of moving toward a shared-care approach for managing patients with prostate problems.

In the light of recent advances, family practitioners need to update and expand their knowledge and skills in the treatment of prostate disease (Fig. 1.2), and their local urologists must be prepared to provide

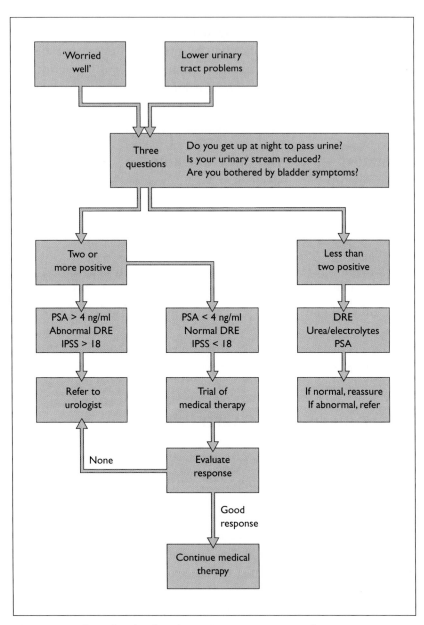

Figure 1.2. Algorithm for shared care. (PSA, prostate-specific antigen; DRE, digital rectal examination; IPSS, International Prostate Symptom Score.)

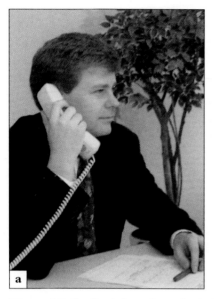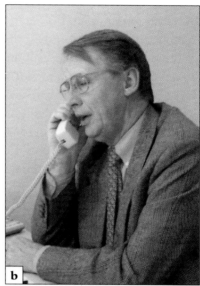

Figure 1.3. Feedback from the urologist is invaluable, especially in the early stages when family practitioners are learning new diagnosis and management procedures.

the relevant help, information and, support (Fig. 1.3). This learning curve can only be climbed by the interaction and cooperation of urologists and their referring family practitioners.

ULTIMATE GOAL

It must be remembered that BPH is a multifactorial disease with varied manifestations, and that prostatic cancer may masquerade as, or coexist with, BPH. In this book, we shall consider to what extent prostate disorders may be safely and effectively handled by the family practitioner, and attempt to identify those patients who should be referred promptly for specialist evaluation, and perhaps surgery, by a urologist.

The ultimate goal of 'shared care' for prostatic disorders is to enhance patient care both by improving understanding of these diseases and by fostering closer links between family practitioners and urologists. Potentially, the rewards of these endeavours may be considerable. Family practitioners will gain satisfaction from improved patient management within their practices, and reduced time and money spent on inappropriate referrals; and, in turn, urologists will be able to dedicate more effort to those patients in whom specific urological intervention can make a significant impact in longevity and on the quality of their life. Most important of all, patients themselves will benefit from an increasingly more efficient and appropriate referral and treatment pattern.

It is appreciated that healthcare provision varies greatly from country to country in terms of the ratios of urologists to family practitioners and the relationships between them. The number of urologists per capita also varies widely (Fig. 1.4). In this book, therefore, we concentrate on the overriding general principles of patient

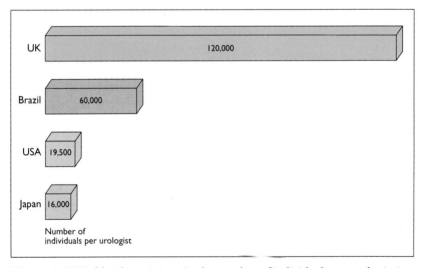

Figure 1.4. Worldwide variations in the number of individuals per urologist in each country will influence the development of shared care for prostatic disease in different countries.

management, rather than country-specific details. However, the final chapter comprises a comprehensive set of case histories that show shared care 'in action'.

CHAPTER SUMMARY

- Many middle-aged and elderly men suffer symptoms of prostate disease that adversely affect their quality of life and yet go undiagnosed and untreated.
- The traditional role in which urologists handle all patients with prostate disorders may no longer be appropriate because of an increasingly elderly population and the introduction of effective medical treatments.
- Family practitioners and urologists can work together to improve patient care – the 'shared-care' concept.
- Clinical BPH may be revealed by asking three questions and quantified by a formal symptom score (e.g. the IPSS).
- Shared care should increase rather than decrease the early diagnosis of prostate cancer and therefore provide better prospects for cure rather than palliation.

REFERENCES

1. Garraway WM, Collins GN, Lee RJ. High prevalence of benign prostatic hypertrophy in the community. *Lancet* 1991; 338: 469–71.

2. Chute CG, Panser LA, Girman CJ *et al.* The prevalence of prostatism: a population-based survey of urinary symptoms. *J Urol* 1993; 150: 85–9.

3. Tsang KT, Garraway WM. Impact of benign prostatic hyperplasia on general well-being of men. *Prostate* 1993; 23: 1–7.

4. Garraway WM, Russell EBAW, Lee RJ *et al.* Impact of previously unrecognised benign prostatic hyperplasia on daily activities of middle-aged and elderly men. *Br J Gen Pract* 1993; 43: 318–21.

5. Garraway WM, Kirby RS. Benign prostatic hyperplasia: effects on quality of life and impact on treatment decisions. *Urology* 1994; 44: 629–6.

6. Brody JA. Prospects of an ageing population. *Nature* 1985; 315: 463–6.

7. Kirby RS, Kirby MG, Farah R (eds). Men's Health. Oxford: Isis Medical Media, 1999.

8. Duncan BM, Garraway WM. Prostatic surgery for benign prostatic hyperplasia: meeting the expanding demand. *Br J Urol* 1993; 72: 761–5.

9. Hennigan TW, Franks PJ, Hocken DB, Allen-Mersh TG. Rectal examination in general practice. *Br Med J* 1990; 301: 478–80.

chapter 2

Extent of the problem

Worldwide, demographic shifts are leading toward an increasingly aged society and, as a result, the absolute numbers of patients diagnosed with benign prostatic hyperplasia (BPH) and subsequently requiring therapy for prostatic disease will continue to rise [1]. In the year 2020, the life expectancy of males at birth will exceed 80 years in many countries, and most men can therefore be expected to live to an age at which they have an 88% chance of developing histological BPH and more than a 50% chance of developing lower urinary tract symptoms (LUTS) caused by BPH. In addition to this, the prevalence of clinical prostate cancer is still increasing [1]. A major effort is therefore required in our increasingly long-lived population to lessen the impact of these prostatic diseases on the men and the women who share their lives.

The three most common diseases that affect the prostate, in decreasing order, are BPH, prostate cancer and prostatitis (Fig. 2.1).

EPIDEMIOLOGY OF BENIGN PROSTATIC HYPERPLASIA

In discussing the epidemiology, it is necessary to distinguish between histological BPH and clinical BPH. Histological BPH is usually determined on the basis of autopsy findings, while clinical BPH consists of three important features: benign prostatic enlargement (BPE), LUTS and bladder outlet obstruction (BOO). As illustrated in the overlapping circles of Figure 2.2, these three entities can co-exist or occur independently of each other.

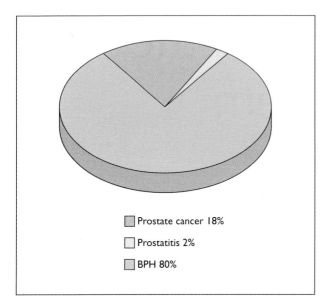

Prostate cancer 18%

Prostatitis 2%

BPH 80%

Figure 2.1. BPH is by far the most common condition in men who present with prostate problems.

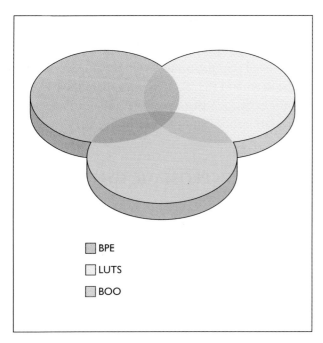

BPE

LUTS

BOO

Figure 2.2. The three fundamental features of BPH – benign prostatic enlargement (BPE), lower urinary tract symptoms (LUTS) and bladder outlet obstruction (BOO) – may occur independently or may coexist.

Prevalence of benign prostatic hyperplasia

The prevalence of histological and clinical BPH, as well as of LUTS, increases with age. Autopsy studies have shown that the prevalence of histological BPH appears to rise from around 50% in men in their 60s to 90% in men over 85 years of age [2]. The proportion of men with palpable prostatic enlargement, however, is rather less, with a prevalence of 21% in men aged between 50 and 60 years, rising to approximately 53% in men in their 80s.

Most important, of course, is the proportion of men who are actually troubled by symptoms. Over the past decade, research on the incidence of LUTS in men has been undertaken in a number of countries. The results from these studies indicate that the prevalence of symptoms increases with age (Table 2.1) [3–7]. These data highlight that the presence of either histological evidence of BPH or palpable enlargement of the gland is not always associated with clinically significant BOO.

A study by Garraway and associates indicates that about half of the men with evidence of obstructive BPH (defined as a prostate [on transrectal ultrasound] > 20 g, and symptoms of urinary dysfunction and/or a peak urine flow rate of < 15 ml/s) reported interference with one or

Table 2.1 International comparison of the prevalence of lower urinary tract symptoms: incidence increases with age

	Prevalence of moderate to severe urinary symptoms (%)		
	50–59 years	60–69 years	70–79 years
Asia [3]	29	40	56
China [3]	24	33	49
Australia [3]	36	33	37
USA [4]	31	36	44
Canada [5]	15	27	31
The Netherlands [6]	26	30	36
France [7]	8	14	27

more activities of daily living (Table 2.2, Fig. 2.3), compared with 28% of men without the condition [8]. In addition to this quality-of-life impairment, many patients reported worry and embarrassment about their urinary function [9].

Another study found that the irritative symptoms (i.e. frequency, urgency and nocturia) were more 'bothersome' and had more impact on quality of life than the obstructive symptoms (i.e. hesitancy, poor stream and post-micturition dribbling) [10]. Despite this definite and measurable effect on quality of life, very few of these individuals had consulted their doctor about their symptoms.

A Danish study has also recorded the reluctance among men aged 60–79 years to consult a doctor about LUTS [11]. Why men do not seek medical help remains unclear, but some of the most likely reasons are shown in Table 2.3. Clearly, there is scope for improving both the level of public education and the knowledge of healthcare professionals in this area. Women, in particular, could be the focus of an educational drive on understanding the disease. In turn they might encourage their partners to consult a doctor appropriately when the need arises.

Effects of race and environment

Although worldwide variations in the prevalence of BPH have been reported, wide disparities in life expectancy may account for some of

---

Table 2.2. Adverse effects of the symptoms of BPH on activities of daily living

Limits fluid intake before travel
Restricts fluid intake before bedtime
Makes driving for 2 hours without a break difficult
Disruption of sleep
Limits going to places without toilets
Limits playing outdoor sports
Restricts outings (e.g., to cinema, theatre or church)

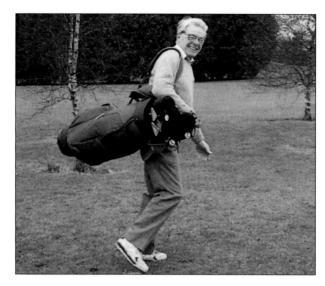

Figure 2.3. Quality of life – a significant proportion of men with symptomatic BPH avoid sport and leisure activities because of their symptoms.

these differences. Clinical as opposed to histological BPH may be more common among black races, but further studies are needed to verify this [12]. Inherited factors have, however, been implicated to explain the high rates of symptomatic BPH reported from the central and northern parts of the Sudan, where intermarriage has often occurred between Arabs and indigenous Africans, whereas no cases were found in the pure African populations of the Southern Sudan [13]. Also in

Table 2.3. Reasons why men with symptoms of prostatic disease do not present to their doctor

Perception that symptoms are a normal feature of ageing
Fear of a diagnosis of cancer
Fear of surgery and its potential side-effects
Reluctance to discuss symptoms with a female family practitioner
Fear of ridicule, and embarrassment of discussing symptoms
Dislike of digital rectal examination
Reluctance to leave the home for diagnosis and treatment

New Orleans, USA, it has been shown that a higher prevalence of clinical BPH occurs in blacks than in whites [14].

By contrast, clinical BPH seems relatively rare in the Far East. In 1900 autopsies performed in Beijing (Peking) over a period of 41 years, the incidence of histological BPH was found to be only 6.6% among the native Chinese and 47.2% in other ethnic groups [15]. The suggestion that southeast Asians who migrate to the USA acquire a higher rate of BPH than their counterparts remaining in southeast Asia points to the influence of both environmental and dietary influences.

Dietary factors

A study from Japan has shown that the incidence of BPH is higher in men who consume large amounts of milk than in those with a high vegetable intake. It has been postulated that certain yellow vegetables and other elements in the Japanese diet, including soya, which are known to contain phyto-oestrogens such as genistein, may exert some protective effect against the development of BPH [16]. A Western type diet, high in saturated fats, may also be associated with a high incidence of prostrate cancer.

Associated conditions

It has also been proposed that BPH is more likely to develop in patients with hypertension. In a study of 326 men with untreated BPH, the incidence of hypertension (systolic or diastolic >140 mmHg and >90 mmHg, respectively) was correlated with American Urological association symptom score [17]. Among men with mild (0–7) , moderate (8–19) and severe (≥20) symptoms the prevalence of hypertension was found to be 15%, 18% and 31%, respectively. Further research is needed, however, to elucidate the relationship between these two common conditions; although it could be postulated that overactivity of the sympathetic nervous system may well be a common factor.

Excessive alcohol consumption may decrease testosterone production and increase testosterone clearance in humans. The effect of alcohol on the risk of developing BPH has been investigated in a number of studies

[18–20]. In two studies a lower incidence of BPH in men who consumed alcohol, particularly beer, was found [19,20]. However, as both studies used BPH surgery as the outcome, the association could be due to the poorer surgical risk of heavy drinkers. Autopsy studies suggest that cirrhosis of the liver may also be associated with a lower incidence of BPH [21]. Theoretically, this could arise from changes in steroid metabolism leading to a relative increase in oestrogen and sex hormone binding globulin, which may in turn protect the prostatic stroma from the stimulatory effects of androgens [22]. Alternatively, reduced testosterone production through alcohol consumption may be a factor.

EPIDEMIOLOGY OF PROSTATE CANCER

Increasing prevalence

Prostate cancer is an important public health problem and one that also seems set to increase. It is the most common form of cancer in men after skin cancer, and is the second highest cause of cancer deaths after lung cancer [23]. The highest mortality rate of prostate cancer is found in Switzerland, followed by Scandinavia (Fig. 2.4). In the USA, prostate cancer is the most frequently diagnosed male cancer, with 334,000 new cases and 41,000 deaths occurring in 1997 [24]. Japan has a low incidence rate, being one-tenth of that in North America [25]. Recent data indicate that the incidence in Japan is rising, however, probably as a result of an increasingly westernized lifestyle [25]. In general, the incidence of the disease is lower in Asian countries than in western countries.

Data from the Olmsted County study indicate that the incidence of prostate cancer and associated mortality peaked in 1991–1992, but has declined in recent years (Fig. 2.5) [26]. Similar results have been reported in the Detroit Surveillance, Epidemiology and End Results (SEER) study, in which a 6.2% decline in prostate cancer mortality was recorded during the period 1991–1995 [27]. These data have been proposed as evidence that PSA screening introduced in the USA in 1991 may have a beneficial effect on mortality rates.

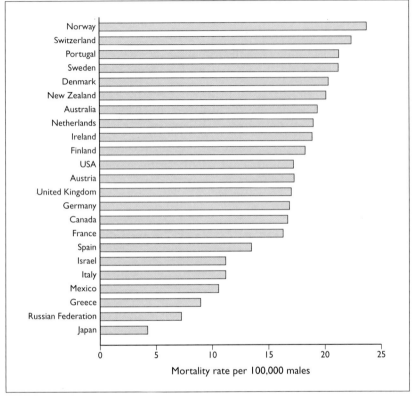

Figure 2.4. Age-adjusted mortality rates by country per 100,000 males [23].

Effects of race

Although relatively few studies have researched the epidemiology of prostate cancer, some facts are established. The incidence of clinical prostate cancer varies widely throughout the world, with the highest rates being seen in northwest Europe and North America, the lowest rates in eastern Asia and moderate rates in Africa. Data from Africa are, however, unreliable and life expectancy is low, which may lead to serious underestimation. Interestingly, the incidence is much higher in areas with a population of African descent, such as the Caribbean and northeast Brazil [28].

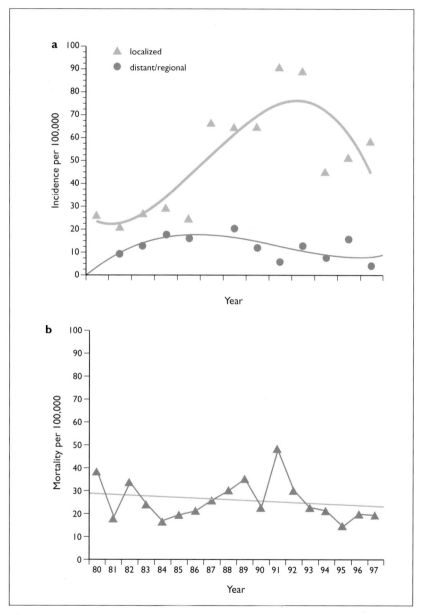

Figure 2.5. Prostate cancer incidence (a) and mortality (b) in the Olmsted County Study [25].

In the USA, the increased risk of prostate cancer in blacks compared with whites is well-documented; the incidence rates among blacks are around 80% higher than those in whites in some areas [29]. Blacks also appear prone to develop the disease earlier and probably in a more aggressive form. They therefore have a higher mortality from the disease [30].

Japanese men appear to have reduced 5 alpha-reductase activity in the prostate gland, which may protect them from developing cancer. The converse is true in American blacks [31]. Thus differences in androgen metabolism, particularly 5 alpha-reductase activity, which converts testosterone to dihydrotestosterone, could partly account for the varying susceptibilities to this disease.

Effects of diet

Migration from Japan to the USA leads to a 15–20-fold increase in the incidence of prostate cancer. Dramatic increases occur in the first and second generations and then level out to match the high prevalence rates of prostate cancer found in Americans. This effect may be related to diet, a theory supported by the observation of an increasing tendency to adopt a more 'western' diet. An increased saturated fat and red meat consumption may increase the incidence of prostate cancer, as it has on other diseases. Attention has been directed to the isoflavenoids, flavenoids and lignans. These products of vegetables, fruit, whole grains and soya are metabolized by the gut microflora into compounds such as enterolactone, daidzein, genistein and weak oestrogens, generally referred to as phyto-oestrogens [32]. It has been postulated that through their growth regulatory activity, phyto-oestrogens may be able to influence prostate carcinogenesis. Suggested but unconfirmed properties of phyto-oestrogens include:

- 5 alpha-reductase inhibition
- Aromatase inhibition
- Tyrosine-specific protein kinase inhibition
- Angiogenesis inhibition
- Antioxidant activity
- Influence E-cadherin expression

- Restraint of the development and growth of animal tumours, but few scientific studies are available to confirm these actions.

Other factors

Occupational risk
The risk of prostate cancer may be increased in men who work with cadmium or in the nuclear power industry [33].

Vasectomy
Although several case-controlled studies have suggested a link between vasectomy and prostate cancer [34], closer scrutiny of these data has cast doubt on this contention [35]. Currently, patients can be reassured that there is no conclusive evidence of a definite cancer risk after this operation.

Genetic predisposition
The possibility of a genetic predisposition toward prostate cancer in some families has been proposed [36]. Individuals who have a first-degree relative with prostate cancer diagnosed at a young age have been estimated to have a 2.2 increased relative risk of developing the disease themselves; those with two first-degree relatives affected have more than twice this risk. Two of the genes responsible for this genetic transmission of risk of prostate cancer are believed to lie on chromosome 1q and on the X chromosome respectively [37,38].

CHAPTER SUMMARY

- BPH is the most prevalent disease to affect men beyond middle age.
- Although clinical BPH is associated with a significant impairment of quality of life, many BPH sufferers are reluctant to consult a doctor, perhaps because of fear of surgery or cancer.

- Prostate cancer is now the second most common cause of cancer death in men.
- As the world population ages, so the burden of BPH and prostate cancer will inevitably rise.

REFERENCES

1. Carter HB, Coffey DS. The prostate: an increasing medical problem. *Prostate* 1990; 16: 39–48.

2. Guess HA, Arrighi HM, Metter ET, Fozard JL. Cumulative prevalence of prostatism matches the autopsy prevalence of benign prostatic hyperplasia. *Prostate* 1990; 17: 214–46.

3. Homma Y, Kawabe K, Tsukamoto T *et al*. Epidemiologic survey of lower urinary tract symptoms in Asia and Australia using the international Prostate Symptom Score. *Int Urol* 1997; 4: 40–6.

4. Chute CG, Panser LA, Girman CJ *et al*. The prevalence of prostatism: a population-based survey of urinary symptoms. *J Urol* 1993; 150: 85–9.

5. Norman RW, Nickel JC, Fish D, Pickett SN. 'Prostate-related symptoms' in Canadian men 50 years of age or older: prevalence and relationships among symptoms. *Br J Urol* 1994; 74: 542–50.

6. Bosch JLHR, Hop WCJ, Kirkels WJ, Schroder FH. The International Prostate Symptom Score in a community-based sample of men between 55 and 74 years of age. Prevalence and correlation of symptoms with age, prostate volume, flow rate and residual urine volume. *Br J Urol* 1995; 75: 622–30.

7. Sagnier PP, Macfarlane G, Teillac P *et al*. Results of an epidemiological survey employing a modified American Urological Association Index for benign prostatic hyperplasia in France. *J Urol* 1994; 151: 1266–70.

8. Garraway WM, Collins GN, Lee RJ. High prevalence of benign prostatic hypertrophy in the community. *Lancet* 1991; 338: 469–71.

9. Garraway WM, McKelvie GB, Russell EBAW *et al*. Impact of previously unrecognised benign prostatic hyperplasia on the daily activities of middle-aged and elderly men. *Br J Gen Pract* 1993; 43: 318–21.

10. Department of Veterans Affairs Cooperative Study of Transurethral Resection for Benign Prostatic Hyperplasia. A comparison of quality of life with patient reported symptoms and objective findings in men with benign prostatic hyperplasia. *J Urol* 1993; 150: 1696–700.

11. Sommer P, Nielson KK, Bauer T. Voiding patterns in men evaluated by a questionnaire survey. *Br J Urol* 1990; 65: 155–60.

12. Rotkin ID. Origins, distribution, and risk of benign prostatic hypertrophy. In: Hinman F, Boyarsky S, eds. *Benign Prostatic Hypertrophy.* New York: Springer-Verlag, 1983: 10–21.

13. Kambal A. Prostatic obstruction in Sudan. *Br J Urol* 1977; 49: 139–41.

14. Derbes VDP, Leche SM, Hooker CW. The incidence of benign prostatic hypertrophy among the whites and negroes in New Orleans. *J Urol* 1937; 38: 383–8.

15. Chang HL, Chan CY. Benign hypertrophy of the prostate. *Chin Med J* 1936; 50: 1707–22.

16. Araki H, Watanabe H, Mishina T, Nakao M. High-risk group for benign prostatic hypertrophy. *Prostate* 1983; 4: 253–64.

17. Pressler LB, Santtarosa RP, Te AE *et al.* The incidence of hypertension (HTN) in a population of men with benign prostatic hyperplasia (BPH): analysis based on the AUA symptom score and race. *J Urol* 1997; 157: 371.

18. Glynn RJ, Campion EW, Bouchard GR, Silbert JE. Development of benign prostatic hyperplasia among volunteers in the normative aging study. *Am J Epidemiol* 1985; 121: 78–90.

19. Sidney S, Quesenberry CP, Sadler MC *et al.* Risk factors for surgically treated benign prostatic hyperplasia in a prepaid health care plan. *Urology* 1991; 38: 13–9.

20. Morrison AS. Risk factors for surgery for prostatic hypertrophy. *Am J Epidemiol* 1992; 135: 974–80.

21. Guess HA. Benign prostatic hyperplasia: antecedents and natural history. *Epidemiol Rev* 1992; 14: 131–53.

22. Robson MC. The incidence of benign prostatic hyperplasia and prostatic carcinoma in cirrhosis of the liver. *J Urol* 1964; 92: 307–10.

23. Parker SL, Tong T, Bolden S, Wingo PA. Cancer statistics 1996. *CA Cancer J Clin* 1996; 46: 5–27.

24. Parker SL, Tong T, Bolden S *et al.* Cancer statistics 1997. *CA Cancer J Clin* 1997; 47: 5–27.

25. Dearnaley DP. Cancer of the prostate. *Br Med J* 1994; 308: 780–4.

26. Roberts RO, Jacobsen SJ, Katusic SK, Bergstrahl EJ, Lieber MM. *J Urol* 1998; 159: 474A.

27. Roberts RO, Bergstralh EJ, Katusic SK *et al.* Decline in prostrate cancer mortality from 1980 to 1997, and an update on incidence trends in Olmstead County, Minnesota. *J Urol* 1999; 161: 529–33.

28. Wilson JMG. Epidemiology of prostate cancer. In: Bruce AW, Trachtenberg J, eds. *Adenocarcinoma of the Prostate.* London: Springer-Verlag, 1987: 1–28.

29. Boyle P. The epidemiology of prostate cancer. In: Denis L, ed. *The Medical Management of Prostate Cancer II.* Berlin: Springer-Verlag, 1991: 3–17.

30. Levine RL, Wilchinsky M. Adenocarcinoma of the prostate: a comparison of the disease in blacks versus whites. *J Urol* 1979; 121: 761–2.

31. Ross RK, Bernstein L, Lobow RA, Shimizu H, Stanczyk FC, Pike MC. 5-alpha-Reductase activity and the risk of prostate cancer among Japanese and US white and black males. *Lancet* 1992; 339: 887–9.

32. Griffiths K, Adlercreutz H, Boyle P, Denis l, Nicholson RI, Morton MS. *Nutrition and Cancer.* Oxford: ISIS Medical Media, 1996.

33. Rooney C, Beral V, Maconochie N, Fraser P, Davies G. Case–control study of prostatic cancer in employees of the United Kingdom Atomic Energy Authority. *Br Med J* 1993; 307: 1391–7.

34. Rosenberg L, Palmer JR, Zeba AG, Warshauer ME, Stolley PD, Shapiro S. Vasectomy and the risk of prostate cancer. *Am J Epidemiol* 1990; 132: 1051–5.

35. Editorial: Vasectomy and prostate cancer. *Lancet* 1991; 337: 1445–6.

36. Steinberg GN, Carter BS, Beaty TH, Childs B, Walsh PC. Family history and the risk of prostate cancer. *Prostate* 1990; 17: 337–47.

37. Smith JR, Freije D, Carpten JD *et al.* Major susceptibility locus for prostate cancer on chromosome 1 suggested by genome wide scan. *Science* 1996; 274: 1371–4.

38. Xu J, Meyers D, Freije D *et al.* Evidence for a prostate cancer susceptibility locus on the X chromosome. *Nat Genet* 1998; 20: 175–9.

chapter 3

Development of prostatic disease

Since antiquity, benign prostatic hyperplasia (BPH) has been recognized as a condition that affects men beyond middle age. Although Hippocrates was probably referring to BPH when he wrote that 'disorders of the bladder are difficult to treat in older men', the first true description of the gland was by Herophilus of Alexandria.

In 1788, John Hunter first noted that the prostate depended on testicular function for normal growth, and he also described the consequences of bladder outflow obstruction due to prostatic enlargement (Fig. 3.1).

THE THREE ZONES OF THE PROSTATE

Almost 200 years later, McNeal demonstrated that the prostate gland is divided into two morphologically distinct zones, central and peripheral, that comprise 25 and 70% of the normal prostatic volume, respectively (Fig. 3.2) [1]. The remaining 5% of the normal gland consists of the transition zone, which lies adjacent to the urethra and extends up to the bladder neck.

Although the histological characteristics of the transition zone and the peripheral zone are similar, the transition zone is the site of development of BPH, while the adjacent peripheral zone is prone to the development of cancer and also susceptible to inflammatory prostatitis.

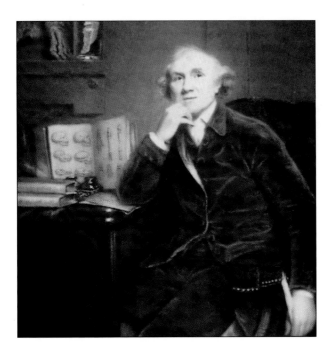

Figure 3.1. John Hunter (1728–1793), one of the fathers of surgery, discovered that prostate growth is a hormone-dependent process.

NATURAL HISTORY OF BENIGN PROSTATIC HYPERPLASIA

In most cases of clinical BPH progression is generally very slow. Proliferation of prostatic tissue with ageing typically leads to prostatic enlargement, which can cause bladder outflow obstruction (BOO); this is manifested clinically as lower urinary tract symptoms (LUTS), detrusor instability, incomplete bladder emptying, urinary infection and, in more advanced cases, by acute urinary retention (AUR). The last condition, AUR, is an unpleasant, painful experience that requires immediate catheterization and frequently requires subsequent surgical intervention.

The longitudinal changes in LUTS related to BPH have been studied in the Olmsted County Study [2]. An 18-month follow-up of 1288 men with mild symptoms at baseline found that 14% progressed to having moderate-to-severe symptoms; at 42 months this figure rose to

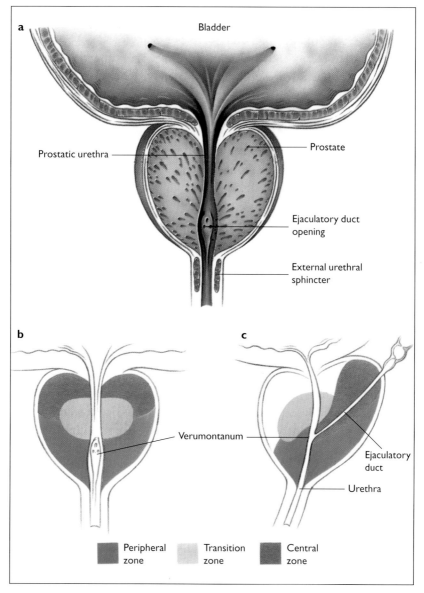

Figure 3.2. Anatomy and morphology of the prostate. BPH develops in the transition zone while cancer more commonly commences in the peripheral zone. (a) Normal prostate; (b) frontal view; (c) sagittal view.

22%. Overall, there was an average increase in International Prostate Symptom Score of approximately 0.18 per year of follow-up.

A 50-month follow-up of 440 men in the Olmsted study showed that the rate of AUR was 6.8 events per 1000 person years of follow-up [3]. The relative risk of AUR was shown to increase with increasing age, with increased symptom severity, with low peak urinary flow rate and in men with large prostates (Fig. 3.3) [3]. Based on these data, it has been estimated that a 60-year-old man with LUTS and prostatic enlargement has a 23% probability of eventually experiencing an episode of AUR.

PATHOLOGY OF BENIGN PROSTATIC HYPERPLASIA

Appearance of microscopic stromal nodules

The first changes of BPH, which may begin as early as the age of 40 years, consist of microscopic stromal nodules that occur in the transition zone around the periurethral area; glandular hyperplasia begins around these small nodules (Fig. 3.4). The nodules may vary in size from a few millimetres to a few centimetres, and are composed of either glandular elements, fibromuscular elements (stroma) or a mixture of both; the smooth muscle containing stroma is generally by far the larger component [4]. In contrast to clinical BPH, the incidence of microscopic BPH does not vary greatly from country to country, and seems equally common in both developed and developing nations, which suggests that the prevalence of microscopic BPH increases with age in all male populations.

Tissue types and obstruction

The proportion of mainly stromal (fibromuscular) nodules to mixed fibroadenomatous nodules varies from person to person, and may help to explain why there is little correlation between prostatic size and the severity of BOO. The degree of obstruction produced by transition zone hyperplasia may reflect the proportion of smooth muscle as opposed to glandular tissue within the stroma. Prostatic smooth muscle is sympathetically innervated and its tone is subject to day-to-day and

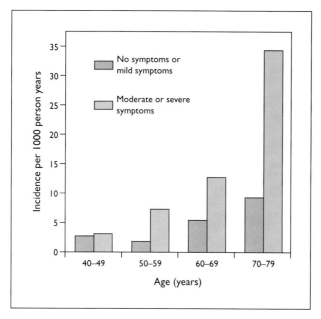

Figure 3.3.
Incidence of
acute urinary
retention by
baseline age and
symptom severity.
Reproduced with
permission from
ref. 2.

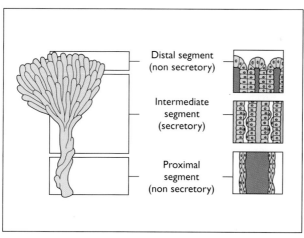

Figure 3.4.
Prostatic ducts
and epithelium.

hour-to-hour neural fluctuation, which may lead to variable urethral compression. In addition, middle-lobe enlargement may lead to a particularly severe ball–valve type of obstruction without much over-all enlargement of the gland (Fig. 3.5).

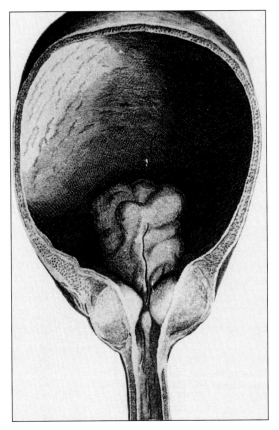

Figure 3.5. Middle lobe bladder outlet obstruction.

The role of prostate-specific antigen

The epithelial cells of BPH elaborate large quantities of prostate-specific antigen (PSA), a protease whose function is to liquefy semen after ejaculation (Fig. 3.6). Low levels of PSA (<4.0 ng/ml) are normally measurable in the serum of all men. Most PSA is bound to serum proteins, such as alpha$_1$-antichymotrypsin; a smaller proportion is unbound or 'free'. The lower the level of 'free' PSA, the greater the risk that the individual is harbouring adenocarcinoma in his prostate. Serum PSA levels may be elevated in 25% or more of patients with BPH and in most of those with significant prostate cancer. Stamey *et al.* reported that the serum PSA value increases by an average of 0.3 ng/ml for each gram

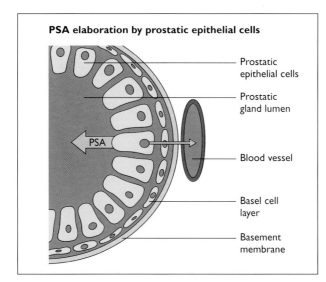

Figure 3.6.
Prostate-specific antigen (PSA) secretion.

of BPH tissue present (Fig. 3.7), which is only one-tenth of the increase that results from each gram of prostate cancer tissue [5].

EFFECTS OF PROSTATIC ENLARGEMENT ON THE URINARY TRACT

Early effects
As the development of BPH is generally slow and insidious, changes within the lower urinary tract occur gradually, which often makes them difficult for the patient, his partner or relatives to perceive (Fig. 3.8). Obstruction to urine flow results from reduced distensibility of the prostatic urethra, which is caused by an enlarging prostate. This leads to a loss of bladder compliance and involuntary ('unstable') detrusor contractions during filling in up to 70% of patients, as well as difficulty in emptying the bladder [6].

As in other smooth muscle systems, the response of the detrusor muscle to obstruction is a combination of smooth muscle cell hypertrophy and connective-tissue infiltration [7]. In addition, the density

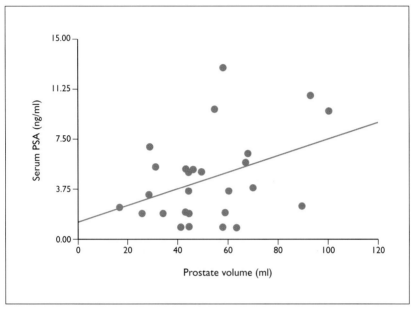

Figure 3.7. Prostate-specific antigen (PSA) levels increase with prostatic enlargement.

of parasympathetic nerves is significantly reduced, leading to a relative denervation of the smooth muscle, which responds by secondary detrusor instability (Fig. 3.9) [8]. Such denervation may explain not only the irritative symptoms of clinical BPH, but also the persistent symptoms of frequency and urgency following transurethral resection of the prostate (TURP), which may occasionally last for up to 1 year after operation. During this time, gradual reinnervation may occur resulting in a progressive improvement in symptoms.

Associated pathology
Patients often tend to ignore the obstructive symptoms of prostatic enlargement, such as poor flow and hesitancy, and are more troubled as irritative symptoms develop [9]. However, these symptoms of

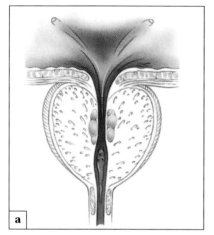
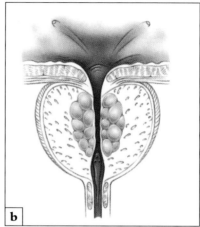
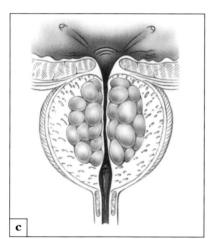

Figure 3.8. Progressive development of BPH. (a) Mild BPH arises just underneath the lining of the prostatic urethra in the transition zone of the prostate. (b) Moderate BPH: as the tissue grows, it encroaches upon and pushes into the channel of the prostatic urethra. (c) Severe BPH: the hyperplastic tissue has replaced most of the true prostate tissue and severely restricts the channel of the prostatic urethra.

frequency, urgency and nocturia, which have been shown to have a greater impact on quality of life, may also occur in the presence of other urinary tract pathology, such as urinary tract tuberculosis, carcinoma *in situ* or bladder stones. Urgent referral should therefore be considered in patients with disproportionately severe symptoms, and especially in those with haematuria or persistent dysuria as these may indicate the presence of malignancy.

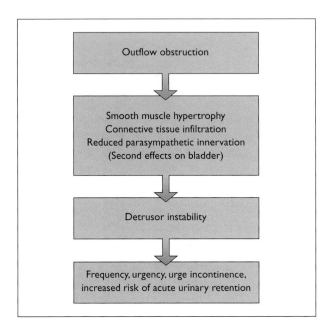

Figure 3.9. Consequences of outflow obstruction.

Late effects

Chronic urinary retention

Gradual overdistension of the detrusor muscle may eventually result in enuresis, as well as in the classic symptoms of BPH; chronic retention of urine should be considered in any elderly man who develops bed-wetting. When massive overdistension of the detrusor muscle occurs, the degree of denervation and associated smooth muscle damage may be so profound that full recovery of bladder function may never occur.

Acute urinary retention

It is unfortunate that so many men still present with AUR despite sometimes having very few preceding BPH-related symptoms. Acute retention is potentially a traumatic life event, and surgery for the condition carries a higher risk of mortality and morbidity than does elective TURP [10]. Severe symptoms, an enlarged prostate, a large volume of residual urine, low peak flow rate, and increasing age are all risk factors for AUR.

Other effects

Long-standing BOO may also result in:

- bladder stone formation
- diverticula formation
- dilatation of the upper tracts with hydroureter and hydronephrosis; over a prolonged period, renal impairment may result and symptoms of uraemia may develop.

Other symptoms related to BOO may occur, including the development of bladder diverticula, urinary tract infection and pyelonephritis (Fig. 3.10). Bladder calculi result in intermittent obstruction, frequency and dysuria, as well as urinary tract infection. The congested

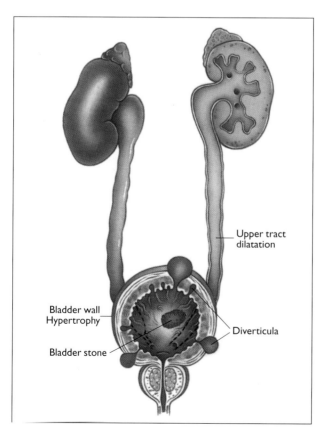

Figure 3.10.
Secondary effects of bladder outflow obstruction caused by BPH.

Upper tract dilatation

Bladder wall Hypertrophy

Diverticula

Bladder stone

vascular bed of the prostate may sometimes lead to intermittent haematuria, which is often maximal on initiation of urination, and must be investigated by intravenous cystoscopy to exclude coexistent transitional cell carcinoma or other urography and urological malignancy.

NATURAL HISTORY OF PROSTATE CANCER

Prostate cancer is a common disease in men above the age of 50 years [11]. More than 80% of all cases of the disease are diagnosed in men aged over 65 years [12], with a median age at diagnosis of 72 years [13]. Mortality from prostate cancer declines after the age of 80 years, but this probably results from competing causes of death. In contrast, survival rates for prostate cancer observed in patients diagnosed before the age of 55 years are lower (Fig. 3.11), which may result from a more aggressive form of the disease in younger men or, possibly, from later diagnosis as a result of failure to suspect the disease in this younger age group.

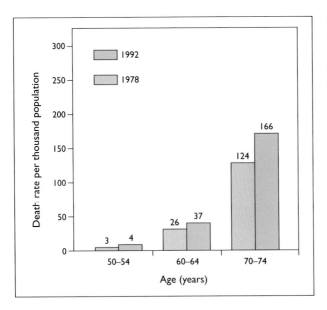

Figure 3.11. Prostate cancer mortality trends have increased in the UK and elsewhere.

Some prostate cancers progress slowly and present little risk to the overall health of the patient. These cancers are almost always small, focal and well-differentiated in patients with low levels of PSA. Most clinically detected prostate cancers are not indolent and do pose a serious threat to health and life expectancy, the obvious exception being in elderly men or those with serious co-morbid conditions.

Data on morbidity and mortality from local prostate cancer progression suggest that the risk for well and moderately differentiated adenocarcinomas is relatively low compared with that for poorly differentiated tumours [14]. The 5-and 10-year survival rates reported for stage T1ac well- and moderately differentiated prostatic adenocarcinomas are 75–87% [15–17]; average local and/or distant progression rates are usually 10% or less [18].

PATHOLOGY OF PROSTATE CANCER

Careful histological studies into the pathology of prostate cancer revealed that:
- 70% arise in the more glandular peripheral zone
- 15–20% arise in the central zone
- 10–15% arise in the transition zone.

Staging of prostate cancer
Clinical classification of prostate cancer can be achieved using the TNM (primary tumour, regional lymph nodes and distant metastasis) system (Table 3.1, Fig. 3.12).

Grading prostate cancer
There are several systems of histological grading for prostate cancer based on the degree of glandular differentiation, cytological atypia and nuclear abnormalities. The Gleason grading system (Table 3.2), which is the most widely used, provides one of the most clinically useful indicators of the likelihood of cancer progression, but is subject to some

Table 3.1 Classification of prostate cancer

Staging	Description
Tumour	
T1	Incidental (impalpable and non-visualized by ultrasound)
T2	Locally confined to the prostate
T3	Locally extensive
T4	Fixation or invasion of neighbouring organs
Regional lymph node metastasis	
N0	No regional lymph node metastasis
N1	Metastasis in single regional lymph node, 2 cm or less in largest dimension
N2	Metastasis in single regional lymph node, more than 2 cm but not more than 5 cm in largest dimension, or
N3	Metastasis in regional lymph node more than 5 cm in greatest dimension
Metastatic disease (M)	
M0	No distant metastases
M1	Distant metastases
M1a	Non-regional lymph node(s)
M1b	Bone(s)
M1c	Other sites

variability of interpretation and sampling errors because of heterogeneity of tissue within the tumour.

The anatomical location of the cancer within the prostate may also be important; transition zone cancers may behave in a less aggressive fashion than those that occur in the peripheral zone which are more likely to invade locally and metastasize.

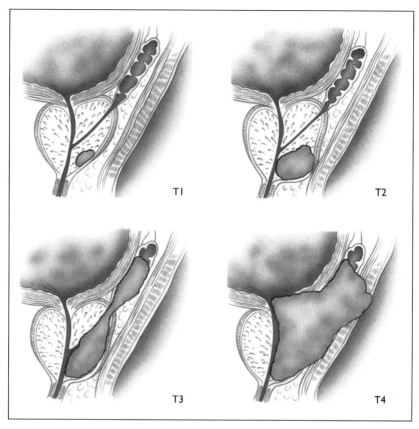

Figure 3.12. Local staging of prostate cancer. The tumour may advance from T1 to T4 with or without the development of metastases.

Table 3.2 Gleason grading system

Grade	Histological characteristics	Probability of local progression over 10 years
Grades 1–4	Well-differentiated cancer	25%
Grades 5–7	Moderately differentiated cancer	50%
Grades 8–10	Poorly differentiated cancer	75%

Predicting the progression of early cancer

At present, those early prostate cancers that progress to infiltrating carcinoma cannot be distinguished with absolute certainty from those that will remain occult within the patient's natural lifespan. Some insight into this dilemma has been gleaned from studying incidental cancers diagnosed at TURP. The median time to progression for T1a (low volume and well differentiated) and T1b (higher volume and moderately or poorly differentiated) carcinomas has been estimated at 13.5 and 4.75 years, respectively [19]. It has therefore become common practice to manage T1a disease in older men by 'watchful waiting' only. Men under 70 years of age, however, often live long enough for clinical progression of the tumour to occur and therefore might be considered candidates for a more aggressive therapeutic approach. Much research endeavour is currently directed towards identifying reliable molecular markers which will accurately predict prostate tumour progression and metastasis.

PATHOLOGY OF PROSTATITIS

Prostatitis is the third major source of prostatic pathology. It is characterized by inflammation of the prostate gland (Fig. 3.13) and presents as both acute and chronic perineal pain. Prostatitis can be divided into four main syndromes:
- acute bacterial prostatitis
- chronic bacterial prostatitis
- chronic abacterial prostatitis
- prostatodynia.

Prostatitis usually occurs in the peripheral zone of the prostate, and is occasionally associated with necrosis, glandular atrophy and abscess formation.

Acute bacterial prostatitis

Acute bacterial prostatitis is usually caused by Gram-negative rods, such as *Escherichia coli* and *Pseudomonas aeruginosa*, and less commonly by enterococci, such as *Streptococcus faecalis* (Gram-positive organisms).

Chronic bacterial prostatitis

Chronic bacterial prostatitis can be distinguished from chronic abacterial prostatitis according to the findings on culture of the expressed prostatic secretions (EPS). It may be caused by a variety of organisms, which include *E. coli*, *Klebsiella* spp., *Pseudomonas* spp., *Mycoplasma hominis* and *Chlamydia trachomatis*. A history of preceding acute prostatitis is not always a feature.

The histological findings show less inflammatory reaction and more focal changes than in acute bacterial prostatitis, and infiltration by plasma cells, macrophages and lymphocytes may be present.

Chronic abacterial prostatitis

Many cases of chronic prostatitis are abacterial, in that no infecting organism can be demonstrated. This condition may be secondary to spasm or to increased pressure in the distal urethra or external sphincter. This pressure may lead to the reflux of urine into the prostatic

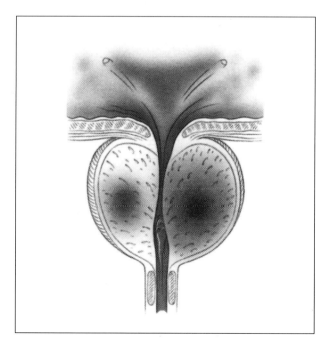

Figure 3.13. Prostatitis. Bacterial or abacterial inflammation involves mainly the peripheral zone and may result in voiding symptoms and perineal pain.

ducts, which results in glandular and interstitial inflammation [20]. Once inflammation has occurred within the gland, it tends to become chronic with periods of remission and relapse.

Pathology of prostatodynia

Pathology of prostatodynia (pelvic pain syndrome) is characterized by pain in the perineum and voiding symptoms, but no demonstrable infection or inflammation.

The cause of this disorder remains elusive, but at least in some patients it may be stress related.

CHAPTER SUMMARY

- BPH develops in the transitional zone of the prostate while both cancer and prostatitis usually develop in the peripheral zone.
- After 40 years of age, the appearance of microscopic stromal nodules marks the start of the development of BPH.
- In BPH, smooth muscle is a more common component of the stroma than glandular tissue; however, the balance of tissues affected varies from man to man, which may explain why prostate size is not related to severity of symptoms or obstruction.
- Serum PSA levels may be elevated in 25% of patients with BPH; unstable detrusor contractions may result in frequency, urgency and nocturia in 70% of obstructed patients.
- Prostatic enlargement caused by BPH can ultimately lead to urinary retention and other serious pathologies. Men with large prostates are more liable to develop AUR.
- The Gleason histological grading system is a useful, though imperfect, predictor of the risks of cancer progression.
- Chronic prostatitis may be categorized as bacterial or abacterial, according to the findings on culture of the EPS. Prostadynia (pelvic pain syndrome) is characterized by a painful but uninflamed and uninfected prostate.

REFERENCES

1. McNeal JE. Regional morphology and pathology of the prostate. *Am J Clin Pathol* 1968; 49: 347–57.

2. Jacobsen SJ, Girman CJ, Guess HA *et al.* Natural history of prostatism: longitudinal changes in voiding symptoms in community-dwelling men. *J Urol* 1996; 155: 595–600.

3. Jacobsen SJ, Jacobson DJ, Girman CJ *et al.* Natural history of prostatism: risk factors for acute urinary retention. *J Urol* 1997; 158: 481–7.

4. Bartsch G, Muller HR, Boerholzer M, Rohr HP. Light microscopic stereological analysis of the normal human prostate and benign prostatic hyperplasia. *J Urol* 1979; 122: 487–91.

5. Stamey TA, Yang N, Hay AR, McNeal JE, Freiha FF, Redwine E. Prostate specific antigen as a serum marker for carcinoma of the prostate. *N Engl J Med* 1987; 317: 909–16.

6. Abrams PH, Griffiths DJ. The assessment of prostatic obstruction from urodynamic measurements and from residual urine. *Br J Urol* 1979; 51: 129–34.

7. Gilpin SA, Gosling JA, Barnard RJ. Morphological and morphometric studies of the human obstructed, trabeculated urinary bladder. *Br J Urol* 1985; 57: 525–9.

8. Speakman MJ, Brading AF, Gilpin CJ, Dixon JS, Gilpin SA, Gosling JA. Bladder outflow obstruction: cause of denervation supersensitivity. *J Urol* 1987; 138: 1461–7.

9. Department of Veterans Affairs Cooperative Study of Transurethral Resection for Benign Prostatic Hyperplasia. A comparison of quality of life with patient reported symptoms and objective findings in men with benign prostatic hyperplasia. *J Urol* 1993; 150: 1696–700.

10. Malone PR, Cook A, Edmondson R, Gill MW, Shearer RJ. Prostatectomy: patients' perception and long-term follow-up. *Br J Urol* 1988; 61: 234–8.

11. Jones GW. Prostate cancer. Magnitude of the problem. *Cancer* 1993; 71: 887–90.

12. Varenhorst E, Carlsson P, Pedersen K. Clinical and economic considerations in the treatment of prostate cancer. *PharmacoEcon* 1994; 6: 127–41.

13. Brawley OW, Kramer BS. The epidemiology and prevention of prostate cancer. In: Dawson NA, Vogelzang NJ, eds. *Prostate Cancer*. New York: Wiley-Liss, 1994: 47–64.

14. Barry MJ. Natural history of clinically localized prostate cancer. *Semin Surg Oncol* 1995; 11: 3–8.

15. Chodak GW, Thisted RA, Gerber GS *et al*. Results of conservative management of clinically localized prostate cancer. *N Engl J Med* 1994; 330: 242–8.

16. Johansson JE, Adami H, Andersson S, Bergstrom R, Holmberg L, Krusemo UB. High 10-year survival rate in patients with early, untreated prostatic cancer. *JAMA* 1992; 267: 2191–6.

17. Maeda O, Saiki S, Kinouchi T *et al*. Clinical study for incidental prostatic carcinoma. *Acta Urol Jpn* 1991; 37: 135–9.

18. Kearse WS Jr, Seay TM, Thompson IM. The long-term risk of development of prostate cancer in patients with benign prostatic hyperplasia: correlation with stage A1 disease. *J Urol* 1993; 150: 1746–8.

19. Lowe BA, Listrom MB. Incidental carcinoma of the prostate: an analysis of the predictors of progression. *J Urol* 1988; 40: 1340–4.

20. Kirby RS, Lowe D, Bultitude MI, Shuttleworth KED. Intra-prostatic urinary reflux: an aetiological factor in abacterial prostatitis. *Br J Urol* 1982; 54: 729–31.

chapter 4

Pathogenesis

Before the recent upsurge of interest in the pathogenesis of prostate diseases, only two factors had been shown to be absolute requirements for the development of benign prostatic hyperplasia (BPH):

- androgen-producing normal testes
- increasing age.

It is now known, however, that a multiplicity of other factors are involved in the pathogenesis of BPH, although androgens clearly play a central role (Fig. 4.1). The multistep cascade of events that takes place from the stimulation of androgen secretion to the replication of cells is being elucidated, and it has been suggested that if a sufficient degree of disorganization of cellular control exists, these events may proceed to prostate cancer [1].

BENIGN PROSTATIC HYPERPLASIA – THE FIVE THEORIES

A number of theories have been suggested over recent years (Table 4.1) for the pathogenesis of BPH, which afflicts most ageing men.

The dihydrotestosterone hypothesis

Dihydrotestosterone (DHT) is the principal intracellular androgen involved with the regulation of prostatic growth [2]. It is formed by the action of the enzyme 5 alpha reductase on testosterone within the prostate [3]. As an androgen within cells, DHT is about five times more potent than testosterone, and it binds readily to the androgen receptors in the nucleus. This promotes a sequence of events to take place within the cell that eventually leads to cell replication (Fig. 4.2).

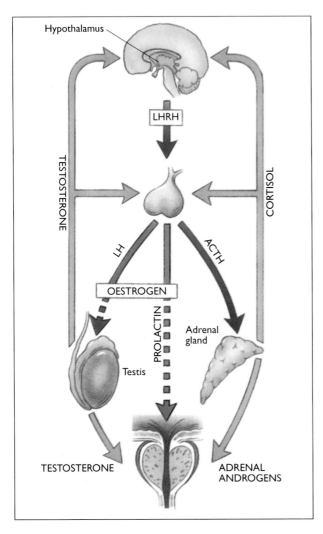

Figure 4.1. Normal control of androgen production and utilization. (ACTH, adrenocorticotrophic hormone; LH, luteinizing hormone; LHRH, luteinizing hormone releasing hormone.)

Early studies suggested that tissue DHT levels were markedly increased in BPH compared to levels in the normal prostate [4]. Although this would have provided an elegant explanation for the development of BPH, these hopes were dashed by further observations. The original studies had compared DHT levels in normal prostates with those in surgically removed BPH tissue. It was subsequently shown that

Table 4.1 Theories for the cause of benign prostatic hyperplasia

Theory	Cause	Effect
Dihydrotestosterone hypothesis	↑5 alpha reductase and androgen receptors	Epithelial and stromal hyperplasia
Oestrogen–testosterone imbalance	↑Oestrogens ↓Testosterone	Stromal hyperplasia
Stromal–epithelial interactions	↑Epidermal growth factor/fibroblast growth factor ↓Transforming growth factor β	Epithelial and stromal hyperplasia
Reduced cell death	↑Oestrogens	Longevity of stroma and epithelium
Stem cell theory	↑Stem cells	Proliferation of transit cells

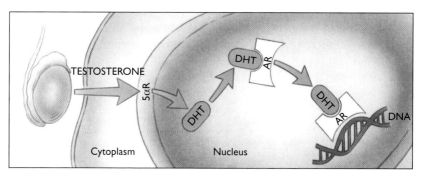

Figure 4.2. The dihydrotestosterone (DHT) theory for the development of BPH. Testosterone produced by the testes enters the prostate cell and is metabolized by 5 alpha reductase (5αR) to DHT. This potent androgen then binds to androgen receptors (AR) and promotes cell growth.

these low levels in normal prostates resulted from autolysis, which could be reversed by incubating the tissue at body temperature for several hours, thus producing similar levels to those seen in surgically removed BPH tissue [5].

Increased 5 alpha-reductase activity

Although the level of DHT in BPH tissue is not elevated, it has been demonstrated that 5 alpha-reductase activity and androgen receptor levels are greater in BPH tissue than in controls. It is the binding of DHT to the androgen receptors that is important in stimulating cell replication, and prostatic cells may therefore gradually become more sensitive to androgens with ageing, because the pathway to increased cell replication involving growth factors, such as epidermal growth factor (EGF), is accelerated.

Oestrogen–testosterone imbalance

The theory that an age-associated imbalance between circulating oestrogens and testosterone plays a role in the pathogenesis of BPH is attractive [6].

With ageing, the circulating level of free testosterone decreases gradually, while the level of free oestradiol remains unchanged. This results in a gradual, but significant, increase in the ratio of free oestradiol to free testosterone. It has been proposed that oestrogens may play a role in the genesis of BPH by sensitizing the prostate to androgens, either by causing an increase in the level of androgen receptors or by decreasing the rate of prostatic cell death. Oestrogens also cause hyperplasia of the stromal cells; oestrogens are produced principally by the aromatization of androgens. If the androgen drive to the prostate is ablated, 'apoptosis' (i.e. programmed cell death) occurs and the prostate, especially its glandular elements, involutes and shrinks.

Stromal–epithelial interactions

Interactions between the glandular and connective tissue elements of the prostate, which are stimulated by androgens but affected by local growth factors, are almost certainly an essential step in the pathogenesis of BPH.

The concept that a form of control of cell growth or inhibition can be influenced by the cell itself or by the surrounding tissues is an essential part of the theory that prostatic stroma affects the growth of the prostatic epithelium. This effect of the stroma on the prostatic epithelial cells has been termed 'epithelial re-awakening'.

Experimental work has shown that the development of prostatic glandular tissue is indirectly controlled by androgens through mediators that arise from the stroma [7]. These are growth factors produced either by the prostatic epithelial cells or by the surrounding stroma. Examples include:

- EGF
- transforming growth factor alpha (TGF-α)
- fibroblast growth factor (FGF)
- insulin-like growth factor (IGF)
- TGF-β (inhibitory).

Reduced cell death

A steady-state appears to exist after the prostate has reached its adult size, whereby the rates of prostatic cell growth and prostatic cell death are in equilibrium. This ensures that neither involution nor overgrowth takes place, so that prostate size is constant. The reduced cell death hypothesis suggests that the increased prostate volume in BPH is a function of a decrease in the rate of cell death or 'apoptosis', perhaps in concert with an increase in cell proliferation (Fig. 4.3). This hypothesis is also supported by the observation that BPH tissue has a lower than normal rate of mitotic activity.

Stem cell theory

Stem cells

It is also possible that BPH results from abnormalities of stem cells within the prostate (Fig. 4.4). A stem cell is a proliferative cell, which rarely divides, but on doing so produces an amplifying cell [8].

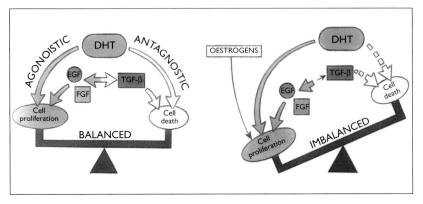

Figure 4.3. The reduced cell death theory proposes that BPH develops as a result of an imbalance of cell proliferation and cell death. (DHT, dihydrotestosterone; EGF, epidermal growth factor; FGF, fibroblast growth factor; TGF-β, transforming growth factor-beta.)

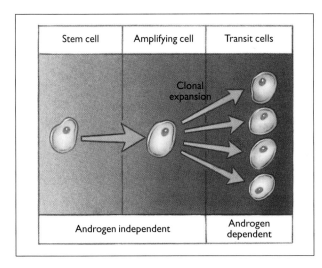

Figure 4.4. The stem cell theory for the development of BPH. Stem cells produce amplifying cells which, in turn, give rise to androgen-dependent transit cells.

Amplifying cells

Amplifying cells proliferate and divide to only a limited degree, but these replications result in a major increase in the total number of cells present. Stem cells and amplifying cells are androgen independent, that is they do not require androgenic stimulation for their maintenance.

Transit cells

A third type of cell, the so-called transit cell, is derived from the amplifying cells; transit cells are capable of only limited proliferation, which is determined by androgenic stimulation. These cells are predominant within the prostate and, because of their dependence on androgenic stimulation for proliferation and maintenance, they undergo apoptosis and disappear from the prostate after castration as androgen support for their structure and function is removed.

Completing the picture

The cause of BPH is complex, multifactorial and involves many steps, both intra- and extraprostatic, and intra- and extracellular. Advances in our knowledge are taking place at an ever-increasing rate, and it will soon be possible to link together the various theories to complete the picture of the pathogenesis of BPH and elucidate its precise relationship to prostatic carcinoma.

PREMALIGNANT LESIONS OF THE PROSTATE

Sometimes patients with ostensibly benign prostatic disease are followed up on a regular basis by urologists. One reason for this is the existence of premalignant lesions in the prostate, which may require extended follow-up by urologists, rather than discharge back to family practitioners.

Prostatic intra-epithelial neoplasia

Prostatic intra-epithelial neoplasia (PIN) is associated with various alterations in prostatic cellular architecture that bridge the gap between a benign and malignant prostate (Fig. 4.5). When these changes are present in pronounced form (so-called high-grade PIN), they require careful follow-up as they are generally considered to be premalignant and carry around a 50% probability of eventually developing into adenocarcinoma of the prostate.

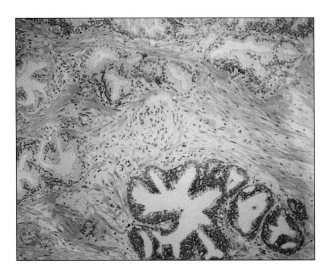

Figure 4.5
Histological section of the prostate showing prostatic intra-epithelial neoplasia (PIN) within the glandular structure.

PIN consists of dysplastic foci of epithelial overgrowth present in the prostatic ducts and acini [9]. It occurs in about 40% of men who are over 50 years of age and who do not have a prostatic carcinoma, but rises to 80% or more in men who do in fact have prostate cancer. Genetic studies of PIN have confirmed that the proliferating epithelial cells share the same types of mutations seen in prostate cancer cells.

PROSTATE CANCER

Although the exact cause of prostate cancer is unknown, recent discoveries link it inextricably to changes in the genetic structure of prostatic cells. Part of the problem in establishing the true cause of prostatic carcinoma is the variability and heterogeneity of the tumour within the prostate gland.

Prostate cancer development is a progressive and multistep process. In the following section a résumé is given of some of the steps that have been recently identified.

Initiation of prostate cancer

It is clear that androgens provide the primary signal for DNA synthesis and cell division within the prostate. This is effected through a complex mechanism, which probably occurs not only in normal prostate, but also in BPH and prostate cancer. The signal is given through various peptide growth factors that stimulate growth and differentiation of prostatic epithelial cells, and also in some cases act as a brake on further growth.

Proto-oncogene activation

Damage to the DNA at certain specific locations can result in activation of proto-oncogenes (Fig. 4.6); these are normal cellular genes involved in the regulation of growth and cellular differentiation. Their activity is also influenced by the surrounding tissues, and the neighbouring cells normally exercise a restraint over the growth of abnormal cells within the prostate.

Cancer may develop when the genetic restraint and control of growth of the cell is lost. This can happen, for example, when oncogenes are activated as a result of genetic changes in the normal proto-oncogenes. Abnormal intracellular behaviour can be induced by oncogene activation or by a change in activity or a change in character of the tumour suppressor genes. It is likely that malignant changes require abnormalities to coexist in more than one oncogene

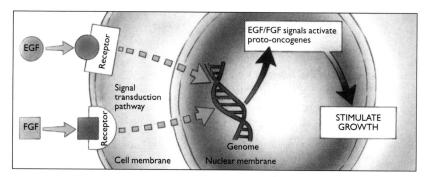

Figure 4.6. The growth factors EGF and FGF activate proto-oncogenes and thus stimulate cell growth.

(e.g. *c-ras*, *c-myc* and *cErbB*). The activation of these and other onco-genes overrides the inhibitory restraints of neighbouring cells and allows tumour proliferation. For example, the activation of the *cErbB* oncogene results in the production of a mutated version of the EGF receptor. This receptor has lost its EGF binding region and signals the need for constant cell division to the nucleus.

Deletion of tumour suppressor genes

The normal cell contains genes that protect the individual against cancer, for example, *p53* and the *Rb* genes. It is known that loss of these genes may result in cancer, and it seems probable that the prostate tumours that occur in younger men, which often appear to have a familial basis, may also result from a specific tumour suppressor gene deletion.

Cancer progression and androgen resistance

If normal growth regulation and control is out of balance, the intro-duction of genetic instability can lead not only to the initiation of prostate cancer, but also to local and metastatic progression.

Angiogenesis

The development of new capillary blood vessels (angiogenesis) appears to be one of the first steps in cancer progression. This may be induced by the abnormal tumour expression of growth factors, such as FGF and other angiogenesis growth factors. New blood vessels not only allow the local tumour to progress, but also promote the growth and development of metastases.

Cadherins and cell adherence

Further progression and eventual metastasis may result because malig-nant cells are less adherent to one another than normal cells. Cadherins are cell-surface glycoproteins required for cell adhesion. Changes in the gene that controls cadherins are involved in progression and metas-tasis and allow the cells to migrate into the lymphatics and the circu-lation [10,11].

Extension of the tumour

Extension of the tumour through the basement membrane and into the extracellular matrix is probably a complex alteration involving integrins (mediators between the malignant cells and the adhesive proteins of the extracellular matrix) and fibronectin (which forms an important part of the basement membrane). If the malignant cell becomes attached, through the mediation of integrin, to the changed molecule of fibronectin, disease progression can occur.

Mitogenic cytokines

Mitogenic cytokines are motility factors concerned with cell movement. If these motility factors (such as scatter factor and migration stimulating factor) deregulate the normal control of cellular migration, this might well account for the migration and metastasis of tumour cells.

Genetic instability

In the growing tumour, genetic instability is an important concept, as it allows the development of cell variants with different degrees of androgen sensitivity. Changes take place that allow the development of androgen-insensitive cells and the death of androgen-sensitive cells. This provides further movement away from the modulating influence of androgens on the growth factors associated with normal cell regulation and the subsequent de-differentiation, a phenomenon known as androgen independence or hormone escape (Fig. 4.7). In patients who exhibit this phenomenon, the prostate-specific antigen levels rises despite continuing androgen suppression.

LOOKING AHEAD

A flurry of activity is currently under way to investigate the mechanics of the regulation of prostate cell growth. These studies focus on the steady progression from normal control through local stimulation to various abnormalities in modulation of these processes and, ultimately, to the development of either BPH or cancer. Improved knowledge of

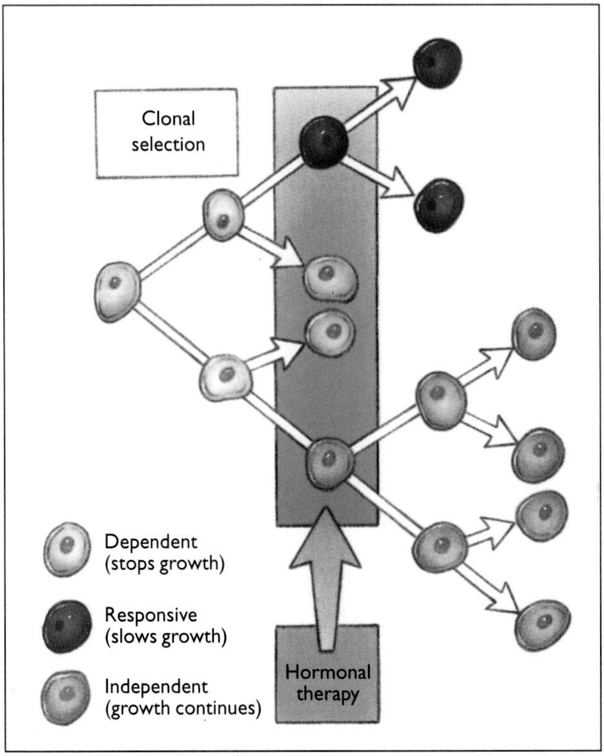
Clonal selection
Dependent (stops growth)
Responsive (slows growth)
Independent (growth continues)
Hormonal therapy

Figure 4.7 Clonal selection: androgen-independent cells are selected out after hormonal therapy and grow to result in 'hormone-escaped' prostate cancer.

the pathogenesis of prostatic disease seems very likely to lead to improved therapies in the future.

Chapter Summary

- The aetiology of BPH is multifactorial and as yet not fully understood; ageing and the presence of androgens are definite requirements for its development.
- The key androgen in the pathogenesis of BPH is DHT, which is produced by the action of 5 alpha reductase on testosterone within the prostatic cell.

- BPH is likely to be related not only to increased activity of 5 alpha reductase and an increased number of androgen receptors within the prostatic cell nucleus, but also to an imbalance of free testosterone and free oestrogen in the blood.
- Other views are that the rate of prostatic cell death and stromal–epithelial cell interactions are important in the pathogenesis of BPH; oestrogens may play a role in such a mechanism.
- The stem cell theory suggests BPH is caused by different types of cells within the prostate that proliferate at different rates as a result of different sensitivities to androgens.
- Prostate cancer development is a multistep process. It may arise from a number of sequential mutations within the DNA of the prostatic epithelial cells.
- Genetic causes of prostate cancer may involve activation of proto-oncogenes and deletion of tumour suppressor genes.
- Vascular development (angiogenesis), cellular adhesion molecules, motility factors and genetic changes that cause apoptosis androgen resistance and metastasis are all involved in the development and progression of prostate cancer

REFERENCES

1. Griffiths K. Regulation of prostatic growth. In: Cockett ATK, Khoury S, Aso Y *et al.*, eds. *The 2nd International Consultation on Benign Prostatic Hyperplasia.* Paris: SCI, 1994: 49–75.

2. Bruchovsky N, Wilson JD. The conversion of testosterone to 5-alpha-androstan-17-beta-ol-3-one by rat prostate *in vivo* and *in vitro. J Biol Chem* 1968; 243: 2012–21.

3. Anderson KM, Liao S. Selective retention of dihydrotestosterone by prostatic nuclei. *Nature* 1968; 219: 277–9.

4. Siiteri PK, Wilson JD. Dihydrotestosterone in prostate hypertrophy. I. The formation of content of dihydrotestosterone in the hypertrophic prostate of man. *J Clin Invest* 1970; 49: 1737–45.

5. Walsh PC, Hutchins GM, Ewing LL. Tissue content of dihydrotestosterone in human prostatic hyperplasia is not supranormal. *J Clin Invest* 1983; 72: 1772–7.

6. Trachtenberg J, Hicks LL, Walsh PC. Androgen and estrogen receptor content in spontaneous and experimentally induced canine prostatic hyperplasia. *J Clin Invest* 1980; 65: 1051–9.

7. Cunha R, Chung LWK, Shannon JM *et al*. Stromal–epithelial interactions in sex differentiation. *Biol Reprod* 1980; 22: 19–42.

8. Isaacs JT. Control of cell proliferation and cell death in the normal and neoplastic prostate. A stem cell model. In: Roger CH, Coffey DS, Cuhna G *et al*., eds. *Benign Prostatic Hyperplasia*, Vol 2 (NIH Publication 87-2881). Washington: US Department of Health and Human Services; 1987: 85–94.

9. Bostwick DG, Brawer MK. Prostatic intraepithelial neoplasia and early invasion in prostate cancer. *Cancer* 1987; 59: 778–94.

10. Giroldi LA, Schalken JA. Decreased expression of the intercellular adhesion molecule E-cadherin in prostate cancer: biological significance and clinical implications. *Cancer Metastasis Rev* 1993; 12: 29–37.

11. Davies G, Jiang WG, Mason MD. E-Cadherin and associated molecules in the invasion and progression of prostate cancer. *Oncol Rep* 1998; 5: 1576–76.

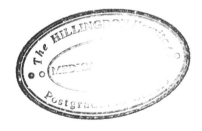

chapter 5

Diagnosing prostatic disorders

In the current era, the diagnosis of prostatic disorders requires a meticulous and methodical approach. Modern testing methods provide useful information that helps to distinguish benign conditions from those more likely to be malignant. Some of the tests may also provide prognostic information about the likely progression of the condition and the risk:benefit ratio of particular treatment options. It is worth bearing in mind the many risk factors for prostatic disease (see Chapter 3) when making a diagnosis and, as always, the first step is to take an accurate history.

HISTORY

Benign prostatic hyperplasia (BPH) is by far the most common diagnosis in men presenting with prostate problems. In practical terms, most cases of clinical BPH can be initially identified by asking three questions (Table 5.1). A positive family history of prostate cancer, especially in first-degree relatives, necessitates an especially thorough screening for prostate malignancy.

Table 5.1 The three questions for detecting prostatic disease

Do you get up at night to pass urine?
Is your urine flow slow?
Are you bothered by your bladder function?

Classic symptoms

Both irritative and obstructive lower urinary tract symptoms (LUTS) are prevalent in ageing men and women. The symptoms associated with BPH can be classed as 'irritative' or 'obstructive' (Table 5.2). Post-micturition dribble is a common symptom caused by pooling of urine in the bulbar urethra, but it is not closely associated with outflow obstruction.

Several structured symptom questionnaires have been developed to evaluate the severity of symptoms and their 'bothersomeness'. Points are assigned for each answer, the sum of which is the symptom score. Early examples of these scores were the Boyarsky [1] and the Madsen–Iversen [2] scores. However, these have now been superseded by the International Prostate Symptom Score (IPSS) [3], which

Table 5.2 Classic symptoms of benign prostatic hyperplasia

Obstructive symptoms	Irritative symptoms
Hesitancy	Urgency
Weak stream*	Frequency
Straining	Nocturia
Prolonged micturition	Urge incontinence
Feeling of incomplete emptying*	
Urinary retention	
Overflow incontinence	

* Correlated most strongly with subsequent need for prostatectomy.

was originally developed by the American Urological Association and recently adopted by the International Consultation Committee on BPH [4].

The IPSS (Table 5.3) is simple and has been validated for test–retest reliability [5]. It can be completed by the patient either before seeing the doctor or during the consultation. However, the correlation between other parameters of lower urinary tract dysfunction (e.g. flow rates and prostate volume) and symptom scores is not always good. Nevertheless, in patients proved by other objective means to have bladder outflow obstruction (BOO) as a result of BPH, the IPSS does give a useful measure of both symptom severity and 'bothersomeness'. Specific symptoms that appear to correlate most strongly with the eventual need for prostatic surgery are poor flow and the sensation of incomplete emptying [6].

The effect that symptoms of BPH can have on a patient varies considerably. An assessment of symptom effect can be made using a quality of life questionnaire, such as the Symptom Problem Index (Table 5.4) [6] and the BPH Impact Index (Table 5.5) [7].

Chronic prostatitis typically occurs in younger men (35–50 years) who present with perineal ache, ejaculatory pain, dysuria and voiding dysfunction. Acute bacterial prostatitis causes symptoms typical of febrile illness, as well as those associated with prostatic disease.

Other important symptoms

Other urinary tract symptoms not included in the IPSS may also be important, although it should be remembered that localized, still curable, cancers of the prostate are usually asymptomatic.

Macroscopic haematuria indicates the need for referral for intravenous urography (IVU) and cystoscopy because of its strong association with transitional cell carcinoma and other urological malignancy.

Dysuria or painful micturition may indicate urinary tract infection (UTI), but may also be the result of carcinoma *in situ* of the bladder. With the latter, urine cytology is often positive for malignant cells; again, cystoscopy is indicated.

Table 5.3 International Prostate Symptom Score (IPSS)*

	Not at all	Less than 1 time in 5	Less than half the time	About half the time	More than half the time	Almost always	Patient score
1. **Incomplete emptying** Over the past month, how often have you had a sensation of not emptying your bladder completely after you finished urinating?	0	1	2	3	4	5	__
2. **Frequency** Over the past month, how often have you had to urinate again less than 2 hours after you finished urinating?	0	1	2	3	4	5	__
3. **Intermittency** Over the past month, how often have you found you stopped and started again several times when you urinated?	0	1	2	3	4	5	__
4. **Urgency** Over the past month, how often have you found it difficult to postpone urination?	0	1	2	3	4	5	__
5. **Weak stream** Over the past month, how often have you had a weak urinary stream?	0	1	2	3	4	5	__
6. **Straining** Over the past month, how often have you had to push or strain to begin urination?	0	1	2	3	4	5	__

Table 5.3 *Contnued*

	None	1 Time	2 Times	3 Times	4 Times	5 or more times
7. **Nocturia** Over the past month, how many times did you most typically get up to urinate from the time you went to bed at night until the time you got up in the morning?	0	1	2	3	4	5

Total IPSS† _____

	Delighted	Pleased	Mostly satisfied	Mixed – both satisfied and dissatisfied	Mostly unsatisfied	Unhappy	Terrible
Quality of life due to urinary symptoms							
If you were to spend the rest of your life with your urinary condition just the way it is now, how would you feel about that?	0	1	2	3		4	5	6

*Adopted from and identical to the AUA symptom score sheet.
†Interpretation of IPSS values: 0–7 mild; 8–18 moderate; >18 severe.
Total possible score = 35.

Table 5.4 Symptom Problem Index (SPI)*

	No problem	Very small problem	Small problem	Medium problem	Big problem
1. Over the past month, how much has a sensation of not emptying your bladder been a problem for you?	0	1	2	3	4
2. Over the past month, how much has frequent urination during the day been a problem for you?	0	1	2	3	4
3. Over the past month, how much has getting up at night to urinate been a problem for you?	0	1	2	3	4
4. Over the past month, how much has stopping and starting when you urinate been a problem for you?	0	1	2	3	4
5. Over the past month, how much has a need to urinate with little warning been a problem for you?	0	1	2	3	4
6. Over the past month, how much has impaired size and force of urinary stream a problem for you?	0	1	2	3	4
7. Over the past month, how much has having to push and strain to begin urination been a problem for you?	0	1	2	3	4

Table 5.5 BPH Impact Index (BII)

	None	Only a little	Some	A lot
1. Over the past month, how much physical discomfort did any urinary problems cause you?	0	1	2	3
2. Over the past month, how much did you worry about your health because of any urinary problems?	0	1	2	3

	Not at all bothersome	Bothers me a little	Bothers me some	Bothers me a lot
3. Overall, how bothersome has any trouble with urination been during the past month?	0	1	2	3

	None of the time	A little of the time	Some of the time	Most of the time	All of the time
4. Over the past month, how much of the time has any urinary problem kept you from doing the kinds of things you usually do?	0	1	2	3	4

Incontinence or enuresis in elderly men is sometimes the result of chronic retention with overflow of urine; however, a low-pressure, 'baggy' overdistended bladder may not always be easy to palpate.

Rapid onset of symptoms and lower back pain may indicate the presence of metastatic prostate cancer, and necessitate prostate-specific antigen (PSA) testing and urgent referral.

PHYSICAL EXAMINATION

Abdomen

To exclude a palpable bladder, the abdomen should be examined carefully in all patients with prostate problems.

Digital rectal examination

Digital rectal examination (DRE) provides the cornerstone of the physical assessment for prostate disease. It is the most simple and cost-effective method of assessing prostate health (Table 5.6), and has almost no morbidity.

To carry out DRE the patient may be placed in the left lateral or knee–elbow position (Fig. 5.1). The normal prostate is about the size of a chestnut and has the same rubbery consistency as the tip of the nose. BPH results in symmetrical enlargement with little alteration in consistency and preservation of the midline sulcus. By contrast, prostate cancer results in stony induration of the prostate that often starts as a palpable nodule and progresses to asymmetry of one lobe of the gland. Eventually involvement and fixation of adjacent structures will occur, especially the seminal vesicles which are normally impalpable.

Rectal examination of a patient with acute prostatitis usually reveals a very tender, sometimes 'boggy' prostate. The findings on DRE in patients with chronic bacterial prostatitis are variable, showing no abnormality, generalized tenderness or localized induration (which may be hard because of calcification or the presence of prostatic stones). The seminal vesicles and epididydimes may also be indurated and tender.

Table 5.6 Clinical parameters that may be assessed by digital rectal examination

Size
Transverse and longitudinal dimension are estimated, as well as posterior protrusion. The normal gland is the size and shape of a chestnut (20 g). With BPH, the gland progressively enlarges to the size of a satsuma (>50 g)

Consistency
Slight pressure applied smoothly while gliding over the surface of the gland to detect whether:
- smooth or elastic – normal
- hard or woody – may indicate cancer
- tender – suggests prostatitis

Mobility
Attempts made to move the prostate up and down or to the sides. A malignant gland may be fixed to adjacent tissue

Anatomical limits
Finger used to try to reach lateral and cranial borders; medial sulcus carefully palpated. The seminal vesicles should be impalpable; induration of these suggests malignancy

As with any manual skill, accurate DRE of the prostate takes a little practice to acquire. The key to mastering the technique is to be gentle, use plenty of lubricant, take sufficient time and think about what you are doing. Even in expert hands, the positive predictive value of a palpable nodule turning out to be cancer on subsequent biopsy is only about 30%, but increases in direct proportion to the rise in serum PSA. It must be remembered, however, that it is quite possible for palpable cancer to be present when the PSA level is normal. Nevertheless, when the DRE is normal and the PSA less than 4 ng/ml, few patients have clinically

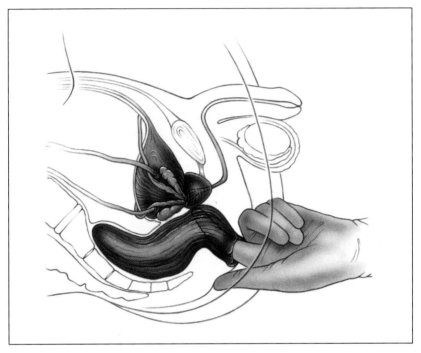

Figure 5.1. Digital rectal examination (DRE) of the prostate should be performed in all patients presenting with prostate problems. Note that only the posterior portion of the gland is accessible to palpation and that size tends to be underestimated with this technique.

significant volumes of prostate cancer present. Note that DRE itself (unlike prostatic biopsy) does not usually cause a significant rise in serum PSA value. The finding of a large, clinically benign prostate may have prognostic significance in terms of predicting the risk of acute urinary retention (AUR). It may also be helpful in selecting the most appropriate treatment options for medical therapy for BPH (see Chapter 6).

It should be noted that DRE underestimates the volume of the prostate, particularly those over 30 ml [8]. The average underestimation compared with transrectal ultrasound (TRUS) measurements was shown to be 9–12% for prostate volumes of 30–39 ml and 17–27% for volumes of 40–49 ml.

INVESTIGATIONS

Urinalysis

Ideally, urinalysis is performed in all men who present with LUTS and, if positive, urine microscopy and culture are carried out to exclude haematuria or UTI. Patients with particularly intractable irritative symptoms should also undergo urine cytology to identify carcinoma *in situ* caused by transitional cell carcinoma, an unusual but important diagnosis.

Expressed prostatic secretions

The diagnosis of chronic prostatitis requires evidence of an excessive number of white (pus) cells in the expressed prostate secretions (EPS) following prostatic massage (Fig. 5.2), or the post-prostatic massage urine

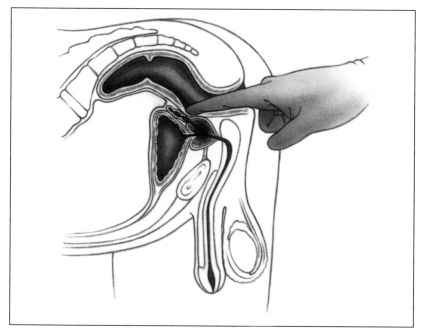

Figure 5.2. Massaging the prostate. Prostatic secretions can be massaged into the urethra and collected for microbiological culture and sensitivity studies.

specimen, above that found in the first voided urine or in the midstream urine (MSU). A positive culture confirms bacterial rather than abacterial prostatitis. Patients with no objective evidence of an inflammatory condition are described as suffering from prostatodynia, the aetiology of which is unclear but may sometimes be psychological.

Creatinine and electrolytes

Approximately 10% of patients with BPH seen by urologists have some degree of renal insufficiency. While the renal impairment does not always result from prostatic obstruction, it may influence the performance of other diagnostic tests, such as IVU, and in itself suggests the need for more urgent treatment. It is therefore recommended that blood urea, electrolytes and creatinine values are determined as a safety check in most patients with LUTS.

Prostate-specific antigen

As PSA (Table 5.7) is so often mildly elevated in BPH, it is an imperfect serum marker for prostate cancer. However, this test does identify a group of patients who are especially at risk of harbouring malignancy. While PSA tests are not mandatory in the evaluation of patients with prostatism, it is recommended in men under 75 years of age in whom the identification of prostate cancer would influence treatment decisions. There is no evidence that DRE in itself increases the serum PSA level significantly and patients may therefore have blood drawn for PSA estimation after DRE during their first visit to the doctor.

Interpreting prostate-specific antigen

If the PSA value is greater than 10 ng/ml, the chance of the patient having cancer on biopsy is about 60% [9]; however, only about 2% of patients with BPH have PSA values above 10 ng/ml (Table 5.8). By contrast, if the PSA is between 4.1 and 10 ng/ml, the risk of cancer on prostatic biopsy falls to around 20% [10]. This is because minor PSA elevations in the 4–10 ng/ml range are present in about 25% of patients with histologically proved BPH, and about 70–80%

of patients with localized, significant-volume prostate cancer [11]. Overall, if the PSA is greater than 4 ng/ml the likelihood of prostate cancer is in the region of 25–30%. A rising PSA may also be an indicator of malignancy (Fig. 5.3).

Table 5.7 Features of prostate-specific antigen (PSA)

Glycoprotein, the function of which is to liquify semen
Produced exclusively by prostatic epithelium
Normal serum value <4.0 ng/ml
Elevated in 25% of patients with BPH
Increased in most cases of prostate cancer
Tends to rise progressively both with age and prostatic volume
May occur in two forms: free or conjugated
Low percent free PSA is suggestive of prostrate cancer
Valuable as a surrogate for prostate volume

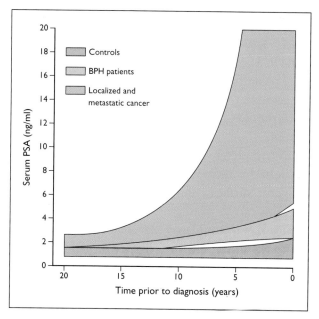

Figure 5.3. Comparison of increases in serum prostate-specific antigen (PSA) levels with time prior to the diagnosis of the prostate condition.

Table 5.8 Interpretation of prostate-specific antigen (PSA) values

PSA value	Interpretation
0.5–4 ng/ml	Normal
4–10 ng/ml	20–30% chance of cancer
10 ng/ml	>60% or more chance of cancer
Rise of >20%/year	Refer immediately for biopsy

It has been shown that PSA is a useful surrogate for prostate size, and that prostate volume is strongly related to serum PSA in men with BPH and no evidence of prostate cancer; moreover the relationship is age dependent [12]. Since treatment outcome and risk of long-term complications depend on baseline prostate volume, serum PSA can be used to estimate the degree of prostatic enlargement sufficiently accurately to be useful for therapeutic decision making, and it is a useful indicator of treatment response as well as an indicator of the risk of AUR.

Percent free prostate-specific antigen

When present in plasma in a concentration of 1 million times less than in seminal fluid, PSA (a powerful protease) is largely bound to one of two inhibitors in the serum:

- alpha-1-antichymotrypsin (ACT)
- alpha-2-macroglobulin.

Alpha-2-macroglobulin completely envelops the PSA molecule and shields all the antigen from the antibody assay, while the ACT shields only some of the antigenic surfaces (Fig. 5.4), and thus the various bound and unbound forms can be distinguished.

Considerable evidence has accumulated that suggests the proportion of PSA–ACT complex in the serum is higher in patients with prostate cancer than in those with BPH. Similarly, the proportion of free unbound PSA not associated with ACT is lower in patients with prostate cancer than in those with BPH [13]. In patients with PSA

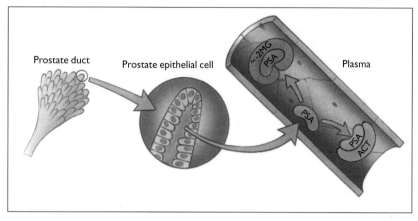

Figure 5.4. PSA is elaborated by epithelial cells within the prostate. In the plasma, it may occur as free PSA or conjugated to either alpha-1-antichymotrypsin (ACT) or alpha-2-macroglobulin (α-2MG).

values between 4 and 10 ng/ml, the additional information of percent free PSA can help as it increases the number of cancers detected and reduces the number of unnecessary biopsies [14]. The probability of prostate cancer for men with total PSA values in the range 4–10 ng/ml can be stratified according to percent free PSA and age (Table 5.9) [15].

Age-adjusted prostate-specific antigen cut-off values

Serum PSA values tend to increase very gradually with age [16]. This is probably the result of slowly developing BPH, but could also occur because more PSA 'leaks' from the prostatic gland lumina into the plasma as the normal cell barriers break down with time. A line drawn through the 95th percentile for PSA values in a population in which prostate cancer had been excluded produced the age-adjusted cut-offs shown in Table 5.9. It has been argued that these cut-off values could serve to increase diagnostic suspicion in younger men in whom a diagnosis of prostate cancer may be more important, because of their longer life expectancy. While such a manoeuvre may improve the sensitivity of PSA testing, it probably does so at the price of reduced specificity.

Table 5.9 Probability of cancer by percent free prostate-specific antigen (PSA) and patient age for patients with PSA levels between 4 and 10 ng/ml [9]

Percent free PSA (%)	Probability of cancer (%)	
	Age 50–64 years	Age 65–75 years
0–10	56%	55%
10–15	24%	35%
15–20	17%	23%
20–25	10%	20%
>25	5%	9%

This raises the possibility of leaving some cancers undiagnosed, but this, especially in older age groups, may not always be undesirable.

In considering the value of PSA testing, it is necessary to judge the ability of the test to distinguish those men who have only BPH from those who also have prostate cancer. In this respect, a single measurement of serum PSA is often inconclusive.

Patients with a PSA level >4ng/ml or percent free PSA <25% and/or abnormal DRE findings should be referred for further study and biopsy unless they are so old, or otherwise unwell, that treatment of any cancer detected may not be indicated. It should be remembered that BPH is at least 10 times more prevalent than clinically significant adenocarcinoma of the prostate.

Uroflow measurement

The measurement of urinary flow rates using a flowmeter is simple, inexpensive, noninvasive and reasonably reproducible. The patient is asked to pass urine into a funnel and a printout is obtained. Although many family practices are not currently equipped with flowmeters, this situation is now changing. Modern flowmeters are unobtrusive and produce

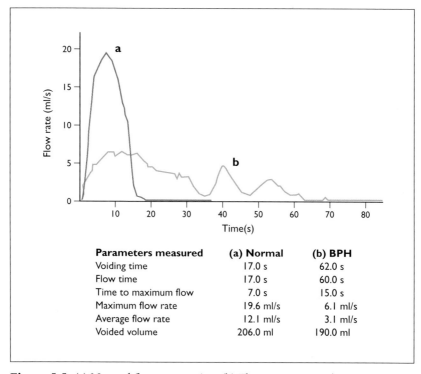

Parameters measured	(a) Normal	(b) BPH
Voiding time	17.0 s	62.0 s
Flow time	17.0 s	60.0 s
Time to maximum flow	7.0 s	15.0 s
Maximum flow rate	19.6 ml/s	6.1 ml/s
Average flow rate	12.1 ml/s	3.1 ml/s
Voided volume	206.0 ml	190.0 ml

Figure 5.5. (a) Normal flow rate tracing. (b) Flow rate tracing showing a reduction in the maximum flow rate in a patient with bladder outflow obstruction caused by BPH.

not only a flow trace, but also a computer printout listing the key parameters (Fig. 5.5). It is, however, important that the voided volume exceeds 150 ml – a requirement that may not always be easy to achieve in a patient with BPH with urinary frequency and a large postvoid residual (PVR) volume. Small voided volumes may give erroneously low flow values. Also, an overfilled bladder may cause abnormal flow readings, especially in patients with severe outflow obstruction.

Maximum flow rate, expressed in millilitres per second, is the most important variable in assessing obstruction (Table 5.10). Maximum and mean urinary flow rates decrease gradually with age and a maximum flow of between 10 and 15 ml/s may be 'normal' in men 70–80 years

Table 5.10 Interpretation of maximum urinary flow rate values.

Flow rate (ml/s)	Interpretation
>15	Normal
10–15	Equivocal
<10	Obstructed

of age [17]. In general, the lower the maximum flow rate, especially in younger men, the higher the probability of BOO, which is predominantly caused by BPH. It must be remembered that the flow rate produced externally is a reflection not only of the outflow resistance, but also of the power of detrusor contraction. Reduced detrusor contractility, therefore, such as occurs in diabetes mellitus due to autonomic neuropathy and also with ageing, may result in a low uroflow. Conversely, an overpronounced detrusor response to mild obstruction may produce a so-called 'high pressure–high flow' scenario. Only pressure–flow urodynamics can elucidate these unusual entities, but patients often find them uncomfortable and sometimes difficult to tolerate.

Measurement of residual urine

As with a suboptimal urine flow rate, an increased postvoid residual (PVR) volume, which is best measured noninvasively by transabdominal ultrasound, may result from either infravesical obstruction or reduced detrusor contractility. Although informative, PVR values vary considerably from day to day and even from void to void [18]. Therefore treatment decisions should not be made on the basis of this test alone. While the test cannot be used to confirm or refute a diagnosis of BPH, it is a useful safety parameter. The fact that patients with large PVR volumes are more likely to develop urinary retention makes them candidates for active treatment interventions rather than watchful waiting. Values of PVR consistently greater than 200–300 ml are a risk factor for AUR and usually suggest the need for surgical rather than medical therapy [19].

Pressure–flow urodynamics

Pressure–flow urodynamics provide the only certain way of distinguishing outflow obstruction from failing detrusor contractility; however, the extent to which they should be used to confirm BOO in BPH is unclear. While flow rate measurement is straightforward, recording of detrusor pressure during filling and voiding requires either urethral or suprapubic catheterization, which many patients dislike. The key parameter of obstruction is the detrusor pressure at maximum flow (i.e. the pressure within the bladder generated by the contracting bladder muscle minus rectal pressure to correct for artefact resulting from abdominal straining). Knowledge of both detrusor pressure and maximum flow rate allows the Abrams–Griffiths nomogram to be used to classify the patient as obstructed, unobstructed or equivocal (Fig. 5.6).

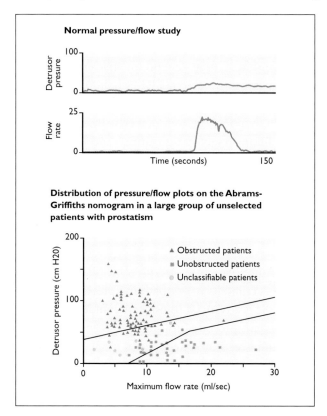

Figure 5.6.
Abrams–Griffiths nomogram.

Urodynamics are, however, invasive and uncomfortable for patients. Current consensus suggests these invasive tests should be confined to:

- patients with equivocal findings in whom surgery to relieve the outflow obstruction is seriously contemplated
- patients in placebo-controlled, randomized trials of new therapeutic modalities for prostatic obstruction.

Transrectal ultrasound of the prostate

In the evaluation of patients, TRUS has two potential values:

- it permits reasonably accurate measurement of both the total gland and the transition zone volume
- it may reveal hypoechoic foci in the peripheral zone suggestive of prostate cancer and also facilitates the taking of prostate biopsies (Fig. 5.7).

It should not be used routinely to assess prostate size, volume or shape in the routine evaluation of men with BPH. However, the success of certain treatments, such as thermotherapy, stents and medical therapy with 5 alpha-reductase inhibitors, may depend on anatomical characteristics of the prostate, making the use of TRUS helpful. Moreover, AUR is more common in men with a large prostate.

On biopsy many of the hypoechoic foci detected by TRUS prove to be nonmalignant, and conversely many cancers are isoechoic or hyperechoic. As its sensitivity and specificity are limited, TRUS is not suitable as a first-line screening test for prostate cancer [20]. It is, however, of great value as a means of guiding the automatic needle for systematic prostate biopsies.

Prostatic biopsy

When DRE and/or PSA abnormalities are present, TRUS provides the most convenient and accurate way of obtaining prostatic biopsies. An automatic biopsy needle is advanced transrectally under ultrasound control and systematic sextant prostate biopsies are taken (Fig. 5.8). It is standard practice to administer a broad-spectrum intravenous antibiotic prior to biopsy and to give a 3-day course of oral antibiotics, usually of the quinolone variety, after the biopsy. The morbidity of

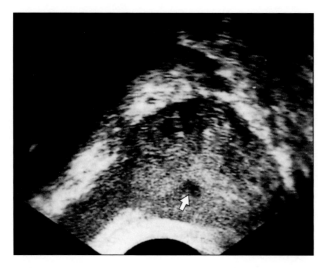

Figure 5.7.
Transrectal ultrasound scan showing a hypoechoic focal lesion (arrow) which proved on biopsy to be a carcinoma of the prostate.

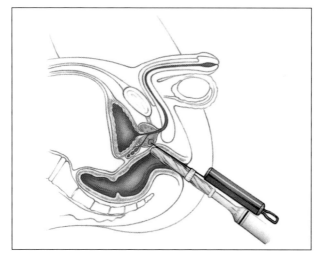

Figure 5.8.
Prostatic biopsy using an automated biopsy gun guided by transrectal ultrasound.

transrectal biopsy is usually minimal, although septic complications may occur up to 3% of patients [21]. Patients should be warned that they may experience haemospermia or haematuria for some days or weeks after the biopsy. Capsular and seminal vesicle biopsies can also be taken in patients at high-risk of extracapsular extension.

Endoscopy of the lower urinary tract

Endoscopy is not indicated in uncomplicated cases of clinical BPH, but does provide information about prostatic proportions (Fig. 5.9), which can prove useful for the application of certain treatment options (e.g. thermotherapy). This information can, however, be obtained more easily by TRUS. Cystoscopy should generally be confined to the investigation of patients in whom concomitant pathology, such as transitional cell carcinoma of the bladder or a urethral stricture, is suspected, not least because the passage of a cystoscope in an obstructed patient may itself induce haematuria or occasionally even AUR.

Imaging of the upper urinary tracts

Imaging of the upper urinary tracts by IVU or ultrasonography is not routinely indicated in clinical BPH, because the diagnostic yield is so low. It is, however, appropriate in patients with:

- haematuria (either microscopic or macroscopic)
- recurrent UTIs
- renal, ureteric or bladder stones
- renal insufficiency.

STAGING PROSTATE CANCER

Biopsy

As in other areas of cancer management, biopsy is essential to confirm the presence of malignant disease. In general, the greater the number of biopsies involved, and the greater the percentage involvement of each core, the higher the probability of extracapsular spread. The tissue cores usually provide sufficient material for the pathologist to give some indication of the degree of tumour differentiation, although not always enough for the accurate assessment of a formal Gleason score (see page 39). It should be noted that prostate cancer exhibits considerable heterogeneity and consequently biopsies may not always reflect

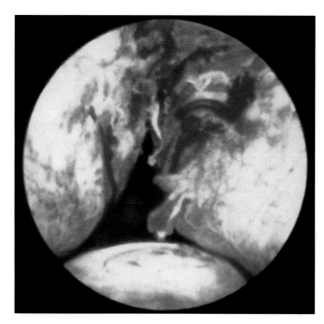

Figure 5.9.
Endoscopic view of lower urinary tract showing the protruding lateral lobes of the prostate in a patient with BPH.

accurately the entire status within a given prostate. Indeed, they often underestimate the stage and grade of the cancer.

Prostate-specific antigen and transrectal ultrasound of the prostate

Serum PSA has been shown to increase with clinical stage, although considerable overlap in PSA values has been observed in all stages. Usually, but not invariably, PSA values above 50 ng/ml are associated with demonstrable metastases. However, serum PSA is not sufficiently reliable to determine clinical stage on an individual patient basis. It can be used in combination with information on clinical stage and pathology from biopsy specimens to predict pathological stage with a reasonable degree of accuracy. Although TRUS results may be informative, scans that provide more anatomical detail often are required to establish whether the tumour is still confined to the prostate, or whether bone or soft tissue metastases have already occurred.

Magnetic resonance imaging

The latest magnetic resonance imaging (MRI) technology with endorectal coils produces exquisite images of the prostate and can sometimes demonstrate extracapsular extension as well as seminal vesicle infiltration (Fig. 5.10). Also, MRI scanning can reveal internal iliac node involvement by a tumour. Disappointingly, MRI has not proved any more accurate than TRUS in the local staging of prostate cancer. In addition, MRI scanning is time-consuming and expensive. Not all patients can tolerate the claustrophobic atmosphere within the scanner, and those with pacemakers, hip replacements or other metal-containing implants cannot be scanned. Intracavity probes allow transrectal MRI scanning, which improves the quality of the image, but makes the test even more uncomfortable for the patient.

Computed tomography scanning

Computed tomography (CT) scans can also demonstrate internal iliac node enlargement, and have the advantage over MRI of permitting skinny-needle aspiration to confirm malignant involvement (Fig. 5.11). Obviously, microscopic nodal involvement cannot be detected. In prac-

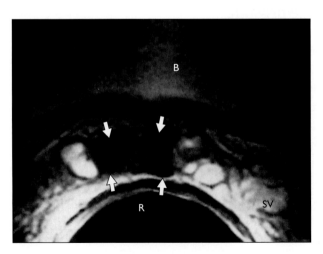

Figure 5.10. Magnetic resonance imaging of the prostate showing seminal vesicle (SV) invasion (arrowed) between bladder (B) and rectum (R).

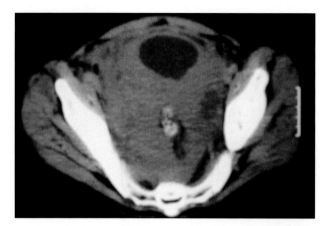

Figure 5.11.
Computed tomography scan of prostate.

tice, CT is considered only when treatment decisions, such as whether or not to proceed to radical retropubic prostatectomy or planning for radiotherapy, hinge on the result.

Bone scanning

Bone scans are an important part of staging prostate cancers (Fig. 5.12); however, they are rarely positive if the PSA is below 20 ng/ml and almost never when it is less than 10 ng/ml. Many urologists still routinely employ this test at the time of diagnosis for definitive confirmation or exclusion of skeletal deposits, but more and more are omitting the investigation in men with very low PSA values and no other risk factors (such as bone pain) for osseous metastases.

GUIDELINES FOR DIAGNOSING PROSTATIC DISEASE

In an increasingly cost-conscious healthcare environment, it is important to avoid uninformative and unnecessary investigations. Although tests must always be chosen specifically for the patient concerned, general guidelines can be given for diagnosing prostatic disease [22, 23].

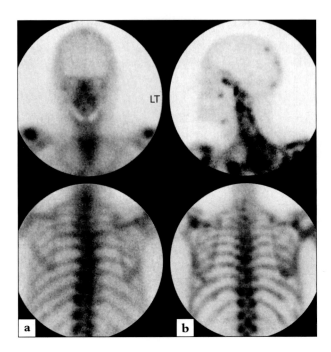

Figure 5.12. Normal bone scans (a) contrasted with positive scans (b) showing multiple 'hot spots' caused by metastatic prostate cancer. This patient's PSA level was 430 ng/ml.

Diagnosing benign prostatic hyperplasia

Patients who present with BOO caused by BPH, identified by case finding or using the 'three questions', or who are seeking reassurance about their prostate should be asked to complete a symptom score sheet (e.g. IPSS), as well as undergo a detailed history and focused examination, including a DRE (Fig. 5.13). Urine should be analysed using the dipstick method and, if positive, an MSU obtained. If a patient complains of excessive dysuria, but the MSU is sterile, urine cytology should be requested to rule out carcinoma *in situ*. Blood should be taken for urea, electrolytes and creatinine estimation; a PSA determination is optional, but recommended in men under 75 years of age after the risks and benefits of the test have been explained. The following findings suggest the need for the family practitioner to refer the patient to a urologist:

- IPSS >18 (especially if sudden onset)
- history of haematuria or recurrent UTIs

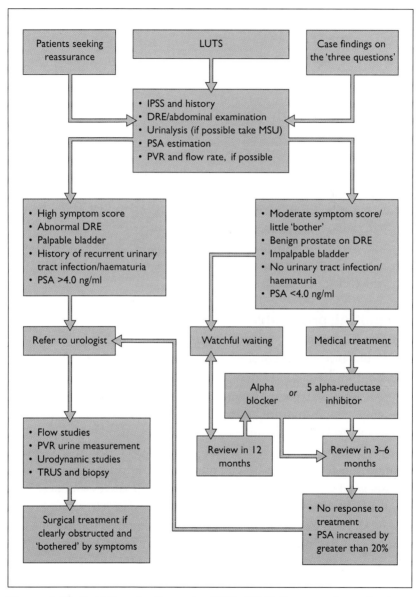

Figure 5.13. Guidelines for diagnosing BPH. (DRE, direct rectal examination; IPSS, International Prostate Symptom Score; LUTS, lower urinary tract symptoms; MSU, midstream urine; PSA, prostate-specific antigen; PVR, postvoid residual; TRUS, transrectal ultrasound.)

- suspicious-feeling prostate
- PSA >4.0-ng/ml
- palpable bladder
- failure to respond to medical therapy.

Diagnosing prostate cancer

Most patients suspected of harbouring prostate cancer can be identified by either a suspicious DRE or a raised PSA (Fig. 5.14). In either (or both) circumstance(s), the patient should be referred urgently for specialist evaluation, including TRUS and guided prostatic biopsy. If the biopsy is negative, surveillance is all that is required. If the biopsy confirms adenocarcinoma, and provided active treatment would be indicated when the patient's age and life expectancy are accounted for, then staging investigations, including a bone scan and sometimes CT and/or MRI scans should be considered.

Diagnosing prostatitis

Symptoms of perineal ache and pain on ejaculation should prompt the family practitioner to consider a diagnosis of prostatitis (Fig. 5.15). Localized prostatic tenderness may be revealed by DRE. The key to accurate diagnosis is the expression of EPS obtained by prostatic massage. A positive culture confirms bacterial prostatitis, and the presence of white blood cells (WBCs) only suggests abacterial prostatic inflammation. The absence of either a positive culture or WBCs suggests 'prostatodynia' – or unexplained prostatic pain syndrome. Acute prostatitis may sometimes be associated with a transient rise in PSA; appropriate treatment should normalize PSA values within 6–12 weeks. Specialist referral for colour Doppler TRUS examination and biopsy should be considered if there is no response to therapy or PSA values remain above 4 ng/ml.

CHAPTER SUMMARY

Diagnosis of prostatic disorders is summarized in Table 5.11.

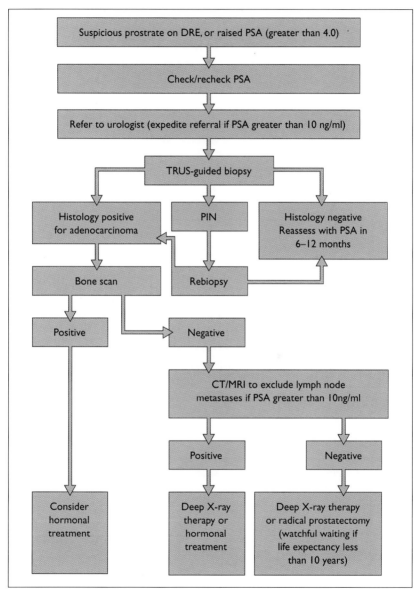

Figure 5.14. Guidelines for diagnosing prostate cancer. (DRE, direct rectal examination; PSA, prostate-specific antigen; PIN, prostatic intra-epithelial neoplasia; PVR, postvoid residual; TRUS, transrectal ultrasound.)

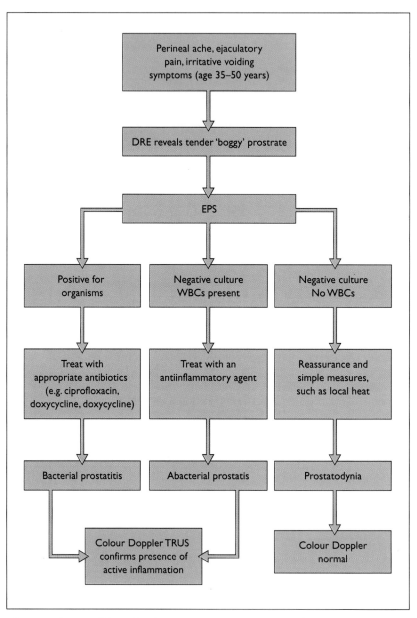

Figure 5.15. Guidelines for diagnosing prostatitis. (DRE, direct rectal examination; EPS, expressed prostatic secretions; WBC, white blood cell; TRUS, transrectal ultrasound.)

Table. 5.11 Summary of prostatic disorders diagnosis

	BPH	Prostate cancer	Prostatitis
Symptoms	LUTS	Asymptomatic until advanced	Dysuria Perineal ache Pain on ejaculation
DRE	Rubbery generalized enlargement	Stony hard induration	Tender 'boggy' prostate
PSA	Normal (75%) 4–10 ng/ml (25%) >10 ng/ml (2%)	>4 ng/ml (>80%)	Sometimes ↑ Normalizes after antibiotics
Uroflow	↓	Sometimes↓	Sometimes ± ↓
PVR	↑	Sometimes↑	Absent
EPS	Negative	Negative	Positive for organisms or WBCs
Urodynamics	↑Voiding pressure ↓Uroflow	– –	– Occasionally ↓ flow
TRUS/biopsy	BPH	Adenocarcinoma	Inflammation
Bone scan	–	Positive if bony metastases present	–
CT/MRI	–	Positive if large -volume lymph node metastases present	Prostatic abscess sometimes visualized

REFERENCES

1. Boyarsky S, Jones G, Paulson DF, Front CR. A new look at bladder neck obstruction by the Food and Drug Administration regulators: guidelines for investigation of benign prostatic hypertrophy. *Trans Am Assoc Genitourin Surg* 1977; 68: 29–32.

2. Madsen PO, Iversen PA. A point system for selecting operative candidates. In: Hinman F Jr, Boyarsky S, eds. *Benign Prostatic Hypertrophy*. New York: Springer-Verlag, 1983; 763–9.

3. Barry MJ, Fowler FJ, O'Leary MP *et al.* The American Urological Association symptom index for benign prostatic hyperplasia. *J Urol* 1992; 148: 1549–57.

4. Cockett ATK, Khoury S, Aso Y *et al.*, eds. *The 2nd International Consultation on Benign Prostatic Hyperplasia*. Paris: SCI, 1994.

5. Barry MJ, Fowler FJ, O'Leary MP, Bruskewitz RC, Holtgrewe HL, Mebust WK. Correlation of the American Urological Association symptom index with self-administered versions of the Madsen–Iversen, Boyarsky, and Maine Medical Assessment Program symptom indexes. *J Urol* 1992; 148: 1558–63.

6. Arrighi HM, Guess HA, Metter FJ, Fozard JL. Symptoms and signs of prostatism as risk factors for prostatectomy. *Prostate* 1990; 16: 253–61.

7. Barry MJ, Fowler FJ, O'Leary MP, Bruskewitz RC, Holtgrewe HL, Mebust WK. Measuring disease-specific health status in men with benign prostatic hyperplasia. *Med Care* 1995; 33: 145–55.

8. Roehrborn CG, Girman CJ, Rhodes T *et al.* Correlation between prostate size estimated by digital rectal examination and measured by transrectal ultrasound. *Urology* 1997; 49: 548–57.

9. Catalona WJ, Smith DS, Ratliff TL *et al.* Measurement of prostate specific antigen in scrum as a screening test for prostate cancer. *N Engl J Med* 1991; 324: 1156–61.

10. Oesterling JE. Prostate-specific antigen: improving its ability to diagnose early prostate cancer. *JAMA* 1992; 267: 2236–8.

11. Oesterling JE. Prostate specific antigen: a critical assessment of the most useful tumour marker for adenocarcinoma of the prostate. *J Urol* 1991; 145: 907–23.

12. Roehrborn CG, Boyle P, Gould AL, Waldstreicher J. Serum prostate-specific antigen as a predictor of prostate volume in men with benign prostatic hyperplasia. *Urology* 1999; 53: 581–9.

13. Stenman UH, Leinonen J, Alfthan H, Rannikho S, Tuhkanen K, Alfthan O. A complex of prostate specific antigen and alpha antichymotrypsin is the major form of prostate specific antigen in serum. *Cancer Res* 1991; 51: 222–6.

14. Morgan TO, McLeod DG, Leifer ES, Moul JW, Murphy GP. Prospective use of free PSA to avoid repeat prostate biopsies in men with elevated total PSA. *Prostate* 1996; 7: 58–63.

15. Catalona WJ, Partin AW, Slawin KM *et al.* Use of the percentage of free prostate-specific antigen to enhance differentiation of prostate cancer from benign prostatic disease. *JAMA* 1998; 279: 1542–7.

16. Oesterling JE, Jacobsen SJ, Chute CG *et al.* Serum prostate-specific antigen in a community-based population of healthy men. *JAMA* 1993; 270: 860–4.

17. Girman CJ, Panser LA, Chute CG *et al.* Natural history of prostatism: urinary flow rates in a community based study. *J Urol* 1993; 150: 887–92.

18. Bruskewitz RC, Iversen P, Madsen PO. Value of postvoid residual urine determination in evaluation of prostatism. *Urology* 1982; 20: 602–4.

19. Dunsmuir WD, Feneley M, Kirby RS. The day-to-day variation (test–retest reliability) of residual urine measurement. *Br J Urol* 1996; 77: 192–4.

20. Terris MK, Freiha FS, McNeal JE, Stamey TA. Efficacy of transrectal ultrasound for identification of clinically undetected prostate cancer. *J Urol* 1991; 146: 78–84.

21. Desmond PM, Clark V, Thompson IM, Zeickman EJ, Mueller EJ. Morbidity with contemporary prostate biopsy. *J Urol* 1993; 150: 1425–6.

22. McConnell J Barry MJ, Bruskewitz RC *et al. Benign Prostatic Hyperplasia: Diagnosis and Treatment.* Rockville: Agency for Health Care Policy and Research, 1994.

23. Roehrborn CG, Kurth KH, Leriche A *et al.* Diagnostic recommendations for clinical practice. In: Cockett ATK, Khoury S, Aso Y *et al.*, eds. *The 2nd International Consultation on Benign Prostatic Hyperplasia.* Paris: SCI, 1993: 269–343.

chapter 6

Medical management of benign prostatic hyperplasia

Shared care is now an increasingly important concept in the management of benign prostatic hyperplasia (BPH) for a number of reasons. These include the increasing prevalence and awareness of the disease and the introduction of several pharmacological agents that offer a safe and effective treatment option for many patients. For shared care to be successful, closer links and more effective interaction between the primary care physician and the urologist are paramount.

Although transurethral resection of the prostate (TURP) is still the established treatment for patients with symptomatic BPH, alternative treatments should be considered for at least some patients for a number of reasons:

- Although postoperative morbidity associated with TURP was reduced during the last decade with improvement in surgical techniques, it still remains at around 10% [1]. In addition, 5-year mortality rates of 17.5% have been reported with TURP, although co-morbidity at the time of operation was high [2].

- Secondly, 10–20% of patients who undergo TURP for BPH require a second procedure within 10 years, either to re-treat the condition, or to treat complications [3].
- The third possible criticism of the acceptance of TURP as the standard treatment for all patients with symptomatic BPH is based on the observation that the prevalence of the disease is much higher than had been suspected [4]. It appears that the number of symptomatic men who present to urologists is only the tip of the iceberg, and that, if less invasive methods of treatment were available, many more men would be more likely to come forward.
- Fourthly, there appears to be considerable variation in the prostatectomy rate from country to country and even within individual countries [5]. In some locations, too many, and in others too few prostatectomies may still, therefore, be being performed.

APPROACH TO MANAGEMENT

Treatment decisions for patients with symptomatic BPH should ideally be made by:
- considering the nature and severity of the symptoms
- assessing the 'bothersomeness' of symptoms and their impact on quality of life
- determining whether urinary flow is significantly lowered and associated with a significant volume of postvoid residual (PVR) urine.

Medical therapy is now a legitimate and safe first-line treatment option with acceptable outcomes. Indeed, the symptomatic improvement achieved by medical treatment is sometimes of the same order as that of TURP, although the improvement in peak flow rates is nearly always better after surgical treatment. Medical therapy is, however, contraindicated in patients with certain specific pathologies (Table 6.1). Medical treatment (Table 6.2) is most often appropriate for patients with mild-to-moderate symptoms of BPH, although patients with severe symptoms sometimes respond well. In

Table 6.1 Contraindications for medical treatment of benign prostatic hyperplasia

Urinary retention – acute or chronic
Renal insufficiency/upper tract dilatation
Recurrent haematuria
Recurrent urinary tract infections secondary to BPH
Bladder stones/diverticula

Table 6.2 Medical therapies for benign prostatic hyperplasia: effects confirmed in placebo-controlled trials

	Agent	Dose	Onset of action	Mechanism of action/effects	Adverse effects
5 alpha-reductase inhibitors	Finasteride	5 mg/day	3–6 months	↓Prostate volume	Erectile dysfunction (3–5%)
	Dutasteride (in trial)	5 mg/day	2–6 months	↓Prostate volume	Probable erectile dysfunction
Alpha-1 blockers	Prazosin* Doxazosin** Alfuzosin** Terazosin** Tamsulosin** (alpha-1$_\alpha$ selective)	2 mg/day q12h 4–8 mg/day 7.5–10 mg/day 5–10 mg/day 0.4 mg/day	2–4 weeks	Relax prostatic smooth muscle Improve symptoms/ uroflow	Drowsiness and headache (10–15%) Dizziness Postural hypotension (2–5%)

*Shorter acting
**Longer acting

our opinion, it should be used as a specific treatment rather than as an interim measure while waiting for TURP. Currently, the main possibilities for the medical treatment of BPH are:

- alpha blockers
- androgen suppression.

Phytotherapy is also used in the management of BPH on an empirical, rather than a scientific, basis in many countries.

5 alpha-reductase inhibitors and alpha blockers have been thoroughly evaluated for safety and efficacy, and certainly have an increasingly important role to play in the management of symptomatic BPH. It is strongly recommended that before starting on this form of treatment the following tests are carried out:

- International Prostate Symptom Score (IPSS)
- digital rectal examination (DRE)
- urinalysis (midstream urine [MSU] and cytology if positive)
- prostate-specific antigen (PSA)
- creatinine
- urinary flow rate.

Both types of therapeutic agent are capable of improving symptom score and peak flow rate, and their effect may in theory be synergic. The value of combination therapy with both these classes of drugs has been tested in three major studies involving terazosin–finasteride [6], doxazosin–finasteride [7] and alfuzosin–finasteride [8] versus placebo. None of these studies has shown any increased benefit of combining the two classes of drugs, at least over a 1 year study period. The men chosen for two of the studies had prostate size less than 40 ml [6, 7], which is not optimal for the activity of finasteride, as the drug has been shown to be more effective in men with prostates over 40 ml [9] in volume.

Follow-up

Patients who are prescribed medical therapy for BPH should be carefully followed-up and reassessed on a regular basis, to ensure that their improvement is maintained and that no other form of intervention is required. Symptomatic evaluation and peak flow rates should be performed every 6 months. Levels of PSA should be assessed every 6–12 months, especially in patients who receive finasteride, which results in a mean reduction in PSA of 50% in patients with BPH, but usually a lesser decline or rise in those with prostate cancer.

ALPHA BLOCKERS

The use of alpha blockers in the treatment of BPH has been investigated in a number of randomized, placebo-controlled, multicentre studies, which demonstrated an early onset of action and lasting improvement in both symptoms and flow rates [10]. Alpha blockers are a safe and effective method of treating symptomatic BPH, with a relatively low incidence of side-effects (Table 6.3). Potential adverse events relate mainly to the effects of alpha blockers on the cardiovascular system (e.g. dizziness, headache, postural hypotension and syncope). Blood–brain barrier penetration can also lead to central events such as asthenia and somnolence. Orthostatic hypotension, which occurs mainly with the first administration of the compound, is a cause of concern as it may result in syncope, especially in elderly patients. Some currently available alpha blockers, such as prazosin and terazosin, therefore need to be started at a low dose to avoid a 'first-dose phenomenon', although newer agents can be initiated at maintenance dosage.

Table 6.3 Effects of alpha blockers

- Gradual dose titration often required
- Improve most lower urinary tract symptoms
- Enhance uroflow by 3–5 ml/s
- Effective in around 60% of patients
- Produce drowsiness and headaches in a proportion of patients
- Result in dizziness and postural hypotension in 2–5% of patients

Symptomatic improvement should be seen within the first 2–3 weeks of treatment and, if not seen within 3–4 months despite adequate dose titration, alternative therapy should be considered. If the patient is found to have significant symptomatic improvement, and an improvement in peak urinary flow, and the side-effects are not troublesome, treatment with these agents may be continued indefinitely.

Mode of action

BPH tissue consists, to a large degree, of an increase in both connective tissue and smooth muscle that is richly endowed with alpha receptors (Fig. 6.1) [11]. This explains how norepinephrine (noradrenaline) can cause contraction of both the prostatic adenoma and of the capsule itself. There is, therefore, a clear rationale for the use of alpha blockade in the treatment of the dynamic component of bladder outflow obstruction (BOO); alpha blockers should improve outflow obstruction by decreasing outflow resistance without interfering with detru-

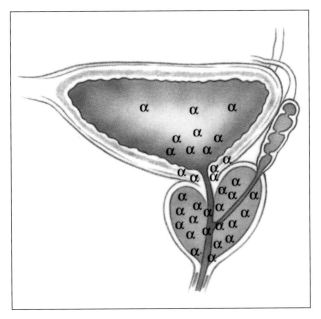

Figure 6.1. Distribution of alpha receptors in the male lower urinary tract. Prostatic smooth muscle tone is decreased by the use of alpha blockers which may lead to improved voiding.

sor contractility, as already mentioned. The newer alpha blockers have improved side-effect profiles, do not need dose titration and are also longer acting.

Phenoxybenzamine

Initial clinical studies showed that nonselective alpha blockers, such as phenoxybenzamine, which blocks both alpha-1 and alpha-2 adrenoceptors, improved symptoms and urinary flow, but were associated with significant side-effects in up to 30% of patients [12]. This led to the introduction of newer alpha-1 selective blockers.

Alpha-1 selective blockers

A drug may be uroselective in that it has a preference for the alpha-1-adrenoceptor in the prostate, or that in an animal model it exerts an effect on the prostate and the urethra without affecting, for example, blood pressure.

It has been demonstrated in the majority of clinical trials that selective alpha-1 blockade can be effective with few adverse events. However, the contribution of alpha-1 adrenoceptors in the trigone, bladder and the spinal cord to lower urinary tract symptoms (LUTS) remains unknown, and their subtypes have not been determined. Uroselectivity defined on the basis of pharmacological or physiological selectivity, therefore, may not be valid from a clinical perspective. Clinical uroselectivity is defined as the desired effects on both obstruction and LUTS related to the adverse events.

All of the classic alpha-1 blockers in clinical use at present appear to be rather similar in terms of clinical safety and efficacy, producing an approximate 20–30% increase in urinary flow rate with a 20–50% improvement in LUTS. It has been claimed, but not proven unequivocally, that the newer uroselective agents have fewer side effects than the older agents.

Interestingly, alpha-1 blockers such as doxazosin and terazosin appear to reduce blood pressure in hypertensive individuals, but have only minimal effects on blood pressure in normotensive patients. In those

20–30% of patients with BPH who are also hypertensive, alpha-blocker therapy may therefore have dual efficacy [13]. These two agents have also been shown to reduce both total and low density lipoprotein (LDL) cholesterol, which may be of value in patients with dyslipidaemia.

Terazosin

Terazosin is one of the most thoroughly evaluated alpha blockers (Fig. 6.2). A study in the USA [15] showed a dose by response relationship for a single daily dose (taken at night) and a reasonably low

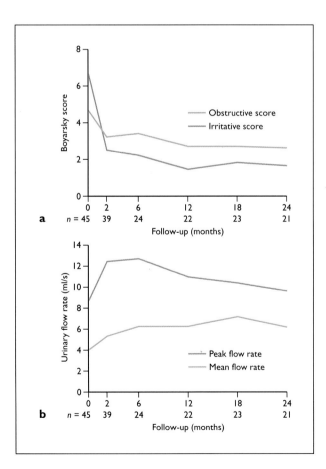

Figure 6.2. Long-term efficacy of terazosin. (a) Obstructive and irritative Boyarsky symptom scores. (b) Peak and mean urinary flow rates. Data from Lepor *et al.* [14].

incidence of side-effects. The dose of terazosin should be titrated up over 1 month from 1 mg/day to 5 mg/day. Occasionally patients may need 10 mg/day. The main side-effects were dizziness and tiredness in about 13% of patients. Terazosin resulted in a statistically significant improvement in both symptom score and peak and mean urinary flow rates.

These results have been confirmed in a 1-year community study involving 2084 men (Hytrin Community Assessment Trial) [16]. Results indicate a 38% improvement in symptom score and a 23% improvement in peak flow rate. Withdrawal from the study because of adverse events was recorded in 19.7% of terazosin-treated patients.

Doxazosin

A number of clinical studies have demonstrated that doxazosin significantly increases both peak and mean flow rates, and produces statistically significant improvements in symptoms [17–19]. The beneficial effects of doxazosin on symptoms and uroflow are seen within the first few weeks of treatment, often before the drug has been titrated to the optimum dose (Fig. 6.3). This has important clinical implications, in that patients may be encouraged to continue with treatment if they experience early symptom improvement. Data also indicate that the efficacy of doxazosin is maintained over a 4-year period [20].

The most frequently reported adverse events reported with doxazosin are dizziness, headache and fatigue; cardiovascular events such as postural hypotension are very infrequent. The incidence of these events does not increase with increasing use. Currently, the recommended dose is 4 mg/day, although some patients may benefit from 8 mg/day. A new, slow-release version of doxazosin is now available that avoids the need for initial dose titration

Tamsulosin

Tamsulosin is an alpha-1A selective alpha-1 antagonist that has a rapid onset of action. Studies show statistically significant improvements in symptom score after 1 week of therapy with tamsulosin 0.4 mg once

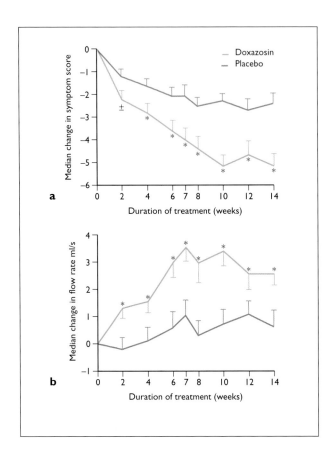

Figure 6.3.
Improvements in (a) symptom score and (b) flow rates with doxazosin. Data from Fawzy et al. [19]. ★Differences from placebo, p<0.005; †significant differences from baseline, p<0.05.

daily [21]. Similarly with maximum flow rate, which is increased to 12 ml/s after a single 0.4 mg dose. Research shows that the efficacy of tamsulosin is maintained in the long-term (up to 5 years) [22]. Dizziness and abnormal ejaculation are the most common adverse events reported with tamsulosin use, but generally the compound is well tolerated and is widely prescribed in many countries.

Alfuzosin

In a randomized placebo-controlled trial [23], a significant improvement in IPSS and peak flow rate (Qmax) was noted in patients

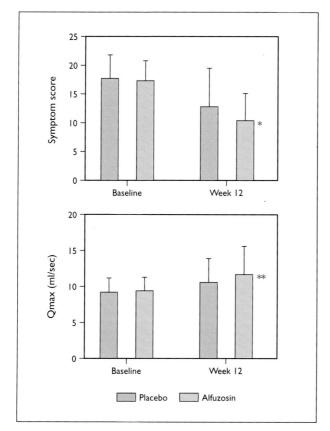

Figure 6.4.
Improvements in (a) symptom score and (b) Qmax with alfuzosin. Data from van Kerrebroeck *et al.* [23]. ★Difference from placebo p<0.002; ★★ difference from placebo p<0.03.

treated with prolonged-release 10 mg once-daily alfuzosin (Fig. 6.4). After 3 months, a 6.9 point (40%) decrease was noted in symptom score, compared with a 4.9 point (28%) reduction in the placebo group (p = 0.002). With regard to improvement in peak flow rate, alfuzosin has been shown to be effective from the first dose. In patients with a maximum flow rate of less than 10 ml/s, mean increases after 3 months of treatment with alfuzosin were 2.3 ml/s (24.5%) compared with 1.4 ml/s (15%) in the placebo group (p = 0.03). In this study, alfuzosin 10 mg o.d. was well tolerated with no clinically relevant effects on blood pressure or heart rate.

Alfuzosin has been shown to reduce the incidence of AUR in a placebo controlled study in men with BPH, although the number of patients was small [24]. It also has the added benefit of restoring normal voiding to a proportion of men with BPH who have been catheterized because of AUR [25].

ANDROGEN SUPPRESSION

Agents that suppress androgen stimulation of the prostate can be divided into three groups:
- 5 alpha-reductase inhibitors
- antiandrogens
- luteinizing hormone by releasing hormone (LHRH) analogues.

Androgen suppression can also be achieved by the use of progestogen (i.e. antiandrogens), such as megestrol acetate and cyproterone acetate, but these are not widely used in the medical management of BPH.

Mode of action

Most patients with BOO resulting from clinical BPH have a considerable increase in the epithelial elements in the transition zone of the prostate gland. The use of androgen-suppressing agents is mainly aimed at this component, although there is also some stromal reduction, and these drugs probably exert their main effect through an overall reduction in prostatic size. The rationale for the use of androgen suppression for BPH is based on a number of observations:
- castration or testosterone suppression decreases prostatic volume and symptoms in patients with established BPH (Fig. 6.5)
- progression to clinical BPH is rare in males castrated before puberty
- in males with a congenital deficiency of 5-alpha-reductase, the prostate remains underdeveloped, but full sexual function is retained [26].

The conversion of testosterone into dihydrotestosterone (DHT) by 5 alpha reductase is a central part of its intraprostatic metabolism, and inhibition of this enzyme would be expected to cause a regression of BPH (Fig. 6.6).

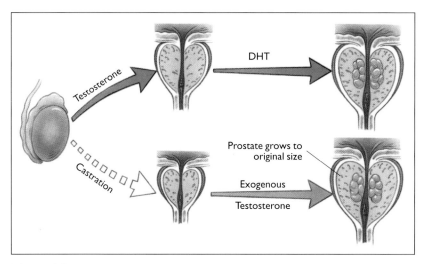

Figure 6.5. The development of BPH is an androgen–dependent process. While castration results in prostate shrinkage, replacement of androgen drive restores the gland to normal and may permit the development of BPH.

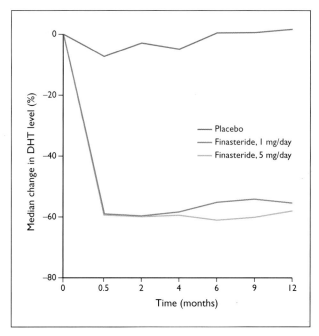

Figure 6.6. Hormonal effect of finasteride. A rapid decrease in serum dihydro-testosterone (DHT) is achieved and maintained for 12 months after oral administration.

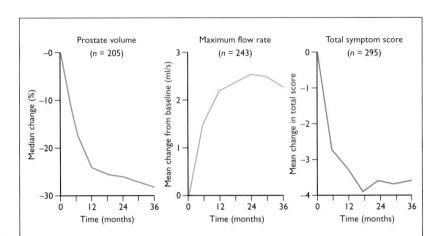

Figure 6.7. Long-term effects of finasteride. As the prostate volume shrinks, the flow rate and symptom score improve.

5 alpha-reductase inhibitors

Finasteride

Finasteride is a 4-azasteroid that has been thoroughly evaluated for efficacy and safety in BPH in many centres throughout the world (Fig. 6.7) [27]. The trials have been randomized, placebo-controlled and continued long-term [28, 29]. Most of these studies concentrated on clinical evaluation by using symptom scores and peak flow rates. The maximum effect of finasteride takes up to 6 months to develop in most patients. Interestingly, a study from Finland showed that positive urodynamic effects on obstruction take place within 6 months of the introduction of the drug [30]. However, therapy for more than 12 months may be necessary to achieve full urodynamic efficacy [31, 32].

Finasteride, 5 mg/day, produces a significant and well-maintained improvement in symptom score and peak urinary flow rate compared with placebo (Table 6.4) [28]. Data suggest that the efficacy of finasteride may be related to initial prostate size. Maximal effects appear to occur in men with prostates over 40 ml in size [31].

Table 6.4 Effects of finasteride
• Effective at 5 mg/day
• Reduces prostate volume by 20%
• Reduces serum dihydrotestosterone by 60–75%
• Enhances uroflow by a mean of 2.7 ml/s
• Decreases prostate-specific antigen by 50% within 6 months
• Results in reversible erectile dysfunction in 3–5% of patients
• Reduces the need for surgery for BPH
• Reduces the incidence of acute urinary retention

Serum PSA values are depressed by about 50% after 6–12 months of finasteride therapy (Fig. 6.8) [33]. Therefore, PSA values should be monitored every 6–12 months and any suggestion of a rise in PSA should prompt urological referral for prostatic biopsy.

Prostate volume is reduced by about 20% in two-thirds or more of patients treated with finasteride. A recent study shows that finasteride reduces the complications of BPH (i.e. AUR and the need for surgery) [34]. Following 4 years of therapy with finasteride, the reduction in risk for surgery was 55% and that for AUR was 57%.

Side-effects associated with finasteride are unusual, the only important one being reduced libido and erectile dysfunction, which occurs in 3–5% of individuals. Some patients also notice a reduction in ejaculate volume. These side-effects are reversible on stopping the medication.

Dutasteride

Dutasteride is a 5 alpha reductase inhibitor that inhibits both isoforms of 5-alpha reductase and is currently being evaluated for activity in BPH. It produces a more rapid and complete suppression of DHT than finasteride and might theoretically, therefore, be faster acting and more effective than the original 5-alpha reductase inhibitor. As yet

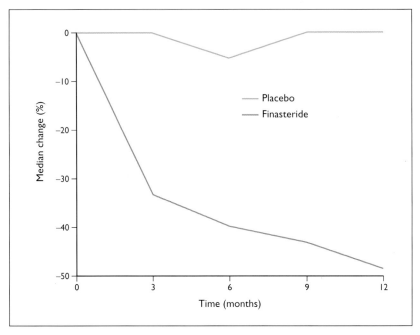

Figure 6.8. A decrease in prostate-specific antigen volumes is observed with finasteride therapy.

there is little published data available concerning its efficacy and safety, although enhanced activity might be anticipated [35]. Phase III studies are currently on-going.

Antiandrogens

Flutamide

Flutamide is an orally active nonsteroidal antiandrogen which competes with testosterone and DHT for androgen receptor sites [36]. Early studies suggest that flutamide significantly increases urinary flow rates [37, 38]; symptom improvement and reduction in prostate size have also been observed [38]. Side-effects reported include nipple pain and gynaecomastia. A more recent combined

European and US multicentre, dose-ranging study on flutamide failed to demonstrate any significant improvement in urinary flow rates or symptom score compared with placebo after 6 months of therapy (J. McConnell, personal communication).

Other antiandrogens

Other antiandrogens studied as potential treatments for BPH include bicalutamide (Casodex®), zanoterone and TZP-4238. One small scale, placebo-controlled study on bicalutamide, a nonsteroidal antiandrogen, reported a 26% reduction in prostate volume, but no significant changes in maximum flow rate or detrusor pressure; symptom score improvements were slightly significant [39]. Breast pain and gynaecomastia were reported in the majority of patients treated with bicalutamide. The other antiandrogens being studied are at an early stage of development. Data strongly suggest that the side-effects of current androgen receptor antagonists outweigh their potential benefit in the treatment of BPH.

Luteinizing hormone by releasing hormone analogues

Analogues of LHRH act by inducing reversible chemical castration in patients with BOO resulting from symptomatic BPH. Most studies of these agents in BPH have been uncontrolled and carried out in small numbers of patients [40], thus limiting any conclusions that can be drawn. Prostatic volume does appear to decrease in patients treated with LHRH analogues, and significant changes in symptom score and peak urinary flow seem to occur. However, the early reports of therapeutic potential for these analogues has not been realized in clinical practice for benign disease. This is largely because LHRH analogues have an unacceptably high level of side-effects, which include hot flushes, loss of libido, erectile dysfunction, loss of facial hair and male habitus. They cannot therefore be recommended at present for the management of symptomatic BPH. One exception is for those patients with AUR and a catheter *in situ* who present with unacceptable risks for surgery. In these cases, this very profound form of androgen deprivation may be indicated.

OESTROGEN SUPPRESSION

Mode of action

Oestrogens are almost certainly involved in the pathogenesis of BPH. Testosterone is broken down peripherally by another enzyme (aromatase) to oestradiol, although the mechanism by which this metabolic pathway can lead to BPH is not absolutely clear. In experimental and early clinical studies, aromatase inhibitors have been found to cause a decrease in prostatic size, but have little or no efficacy in improving symptoms or uroflow in men with symptomatic BPH.

Current investigations

A large clinical trial using the aromatase inhibitor atamestane has been undertaken. Results from a randomized, placebo-controlled trial of atamestane involving 160 patients indicate a 40% reduction in serum oestradiol and a 60% reduction in oestrone, but no significant improvement in uroflow, symptoms or prostate size [41]. A more recent multicentre study showed that reductions in serum oestrogen levels caused by atamestane did not translate into improvements in clinically established BPH [42].

PHYTOTHERAPY

Alternative medical treatments for BPH include mainly phytotherapeutic preparations (Table 6.5) and derivatives of polyene substances. In some countries, phytotherapy is regarded as a legitimate drug treatment, while in others it is considered a dietary nutritional supplement (and therefore not strictly regulated). Most phytotherapeutic preparations are plant extracts that contain different components and are manufactured by different extraction procedures; this prevents a comparison of various preparations. Progress has been made towards isolating individual components (Table 6.6) and identifying their mechanism of action. It remains to be established, however, which of these actions demonstrated *in vitro* might be responsible for any clinical activity.

Table 6.5 Origin of plant extracts used in the management of benign prostatic hyperplasia

- *Hypoxis rooperi* (South African star-grass)
- *Urtica* spp. (Stinging nettle)
- *Sabal serrulatum* (Dwarf palm)
- *Serenoa repens B* (American dwarf palm)
- *Cucurbita pepo* (Pumpkin seed)
- *Pygeum africanum* (African plum)
- *Populus tremula* (Aspen)
- *Echinacea purpurea* (Purple coneflower)
- *Secale cereale* (Rye)

Table 6.6 Components of plant extracts

Phytosterols	Lupenone	Polysaccharides
β-sitosterol	Lupenol	Flavonoids
Campesterol	Terpenoids	Phyto-oestrogens
Stigmasterol	Fatty acids	Coumestrol
	Lectins	Genistein
	Plant oils	

A number of short-term randomized trials suggest clinical efficacy for some preparations [43–46]. Extracts from the plant *Hypoxis rooperi* (Harzol), which contain mainly β-sitosterol, produced significant improvements in symptom score, peak flow rate and residual urine compared with placebo in a 6-month randomized study involving 200 patients [43].

A recent randomized, double-blind multicentre study involving 1098 patients compared the efficacy of Permixon® with finasteride over a 6-month period [47]. Results showed that Permixon® was as effective as finasteride in terms of improvement in symptoms and increase in maximum urinary flow rate. However, the lack of a placebo control and the inclusion of men with smaller prostates, for which finasteride may not be the optimal treatment, are important criticisms of this study.

MANAGING PROSTATITIS

Acute prostatitis

The treatment of acute prostatitis is usually straightforward, and all patients should be started on a prolonged course of an antibiotic active against Gram-negative organisms, such as ciprofloxacin, until the culture and sensitivity tests are available. Follow-up cultures must be carried out to ensure that complete eradication of the causative organism has occurred. A severe infection may lead to urinary retention which may occasionally require suprapubic drainage. Urinary retention usually resolves without the need for further surgical intervention, since the condition responds well to antibiotic therapy. Occasionally, abscess formation occurs and this may rupture spontaneously into the urethra or require drainage transurethrally.

Chronic prostatitis

Chronic abacterial prostatitis may respond to anti-inflammatory agents alone, but bacterial prostatic infections require long-term (3-month) courses of antibiotics. Not all antibiotics are, however, capable of achieving satisfactory bactericidal levels within the gland [48, 49], and the best agent to use is one of the newer aminoquinolones, such as ciprofloxacin or norfloxacin. If this fails, the continuous use of low-dose daily suppressive therapy with an appropriate oral agent, such as nitrofurantoin, trimethoprim plus sulfamethoxazole or ciprofloxacin, may sometimes help. Irritative symptoms may respond to the use of nonsteroidal anti-inflammatory drugs.

Following therapy, expressed prostatic secretions should become negative on culture and PSA values should fall to within the normal range. Failure of PSA values to decline 3 months after adequate therapy should prompt referral for prostatic biopsy guided by transrectal ultrasound to exclude prostatic cancer.

Prostatodynia

A multidisciplinary approach is helpful, which may involve a treatment team that includes a pain specialist, neurologist, physiotherapist and psychologist or psychiatrist. A trial of alpha-blocking agents or striated muscle relaxants, such as diazepam, may sometimes be helpful in treating prostatodynia, but lifestyle changes to reduce stress and anxiety may be more effective. Repeated prostatic massage has been reported to be beneficial. Many of the symptoms are psychogenic rather than physical in nature, and any invasive therapy should generally be avoided.

CHAPTER SUMMARY

- Before prescribing medical therapy for BPH, patients should be fully evaluated by symptom score (IPSS), urinalysis, urinary flow rate, DRE, PSA, serum creatinine and, ideally, determination of PVR urine volume. Only a full pressure–flow urodynamic study will definitely indicate the presence of obstruction, but it is not practical or desirable to carry out this test in every patient.
- Medical therapy is an established treatment option for patients with mild-to-moderate symptoms of BPH. The main options are 5 alpha-reductase inhibitors and alpha blockers. Men with large prostates (>40 ml) may be better suited to treatment with a 5 alpha-reductase inhibitor, such as finasteride, because of their increased risk of AUR. Conversely, alpha blockers are effective in most men with clinical BPH regardless of prostrate size.

- The other forms of medical treatment, such as androgen suppression or aromatase inhibition, do not have a significant role in the management of symptomatic BPH because of their high incidence of side-effects.
- Phytotherapy is considered a therapeutic option for BPH by some investigators. Clinical studies are promising, but further confirmatory work is needed in the form of properly conducted randomized controlled trials in sufficient numbers of patients.

REFERENCES

1.   Uchida T, Ohori M, Soh S *et al.* Factors influencing morbidity in patients undergoing transurethral resection of the prostate. *Urology* 1999; 53: 98–105.

2.   Concato J, Horowitz RI, Feinstein AR, Elmore JG, Schiff SF. Problems of comorbidity in mortality after prostatectomy. *JAMA* 1992; 267: 1077–82.

3.   Roos NP, Wennberg JE, Malenka DJ *et al.* Mortality and reoperation after open and transurethral resection of the prostate for benign prostatic hyperplasia. *N Engl J Med* 1989; 320: 1120–4.

4.   Garraway WM, Collins GN, Lee RJ. High prevalence of benign prostatic hypertrophy in the community. *Lancet* 1991; 488: 469–71.

5.   Wennberg JE, Mulley AF, Hanley D *et al.* An assessment of prostatectomy for benign urinary tract obstruction. Geographic variations and the evaluation of medical outcomes. *JAMA* 1988; 259: 3027–30.

6.   Lepor H, Williford WO, Barry MJ *et al.* The efficacy of terazosin, finasteride, or both in benign prostatic hyperplasia. *N Engl J Med* 1996; 335: 533–9.

7.   Kirby RS, Altwein E, Bartsch G *et al.* Results of the PREDICT (Prospective European Doxazosin and Combination Therapy) trial. *J Urol* 1999; 161(Suppl. 4): 266.

8.   Debruyne FMJ, Jardin A, Colloi D *et al.* Sustained-release alfuzosin, finasteride and the combination of both in the treatment of benign prostatic hyperplasia. *Eur Urol* 1998; 34: 169–75.

9.   Boyle P, Gould AL, Roehrborn CG. Prostate volume predicts outcome of treatment of benign prostatic hyperplasia with finasteride: meta-analysis of randomized clinical trials. *Urology* 1996; 48: 398–405.

10. Kirby RS, Pool JL. Alpha adrenoceptor blockade in the treatment of benign prostatic hyperplasia: past, present and future. *Br J Urol* 1997; 80: 521–32.

11. Shapiro E, Lepor H. Alpha adrenergic receptors in hyperplasic human prostate: identification and characterization using 3H rauwolsine. *J Urol* 1992; 135: 1038–41.

12. Caine M, Perlerg S, Meretyk S. A placebo-controlled double-blind study of the effect of phenoxybenzamine in benign prostatic obstruction. *Br J Urol* 1978; 50: 551–4.

13. Kirby RS, Chapple CR, Christmas TJ. Doxazosin: minimal blood pressure effects in normotensive BPH patients. *J Urol* 1993; 149: 434A.

14. Lepor H, Meretyk S, Knapp-Maloney. The safety, efficacy and compliance of terazosin therapy for benign prostatic hyperplasia. *J Urol* 1992; 147: 1554–7.

15. Lepor H, Auerbach S, Puras-Baez A *et al.* A randomised, placebo-controlled multicentre study of the efficacy and safety of terazosin in the treatment of benign prostatic hyperplasia. *J Urol* 1992; 148: 1467–74.

16. Roehrborn CG, Oesterling JE, Auerbach S *et al.* The Hytrin Community Assessment Trial study: a one-year study of terazosin versus placebo in the treatment of men with symptomatic benign prostatic hyperplasia. HYCAT Investigator Group. *Urology* 1996; 47: 159–68.

17. Chapple CR, Carter P, Christmas TJ *et al.* A three month double-blind study of doxazosin as treatment for benign prostatic bladder outlet obstruction. *Br J Urol* 1994; 74: 50–6.

18. Gillenwater JY, Conn RL, Chrysant SG *et al.* Doxazosin for the treatment of benign prostatic hyperplasia in patients with mild to moderate essential hypertension: a double-blind, placebo-controlled, dose–response multicenter study. *J Urol* 1995; 154: 110–5.

19. Fawzy A, Braun K, Lewis GP *et al.* Doxazosin in the treatment of benign prostatic hyperplasia in normotensive patients: a multicentre study. *J Urol* 1995; 154: 105–10.

20. Lepor H, Kaplan SA, Klimberg I et al. Doxazosin for benign prostatic hyperplasia: long term efficacy and safety in hypertensive and normotensive patients. *J Urol* 1997; 157: 525–30.

21. Barry NJ, Fowler FJ, O'Leary MP *et al.* The American Urological Association symptom index for benign prostatic hyperplasia. *J Urol* 1992; 148: 1549–57.

22. Schulman CC, Denis L, Jonas U *et al.* Tamsulosin, the first prostate-selective α_{1A}-adrenoceptor antagonist: an interim analysis of a multinational, multicentre, open-label study assessing the long-term efficacy and safety in patients with benign prostatic obstruction (symptomatic BPH). *Eur Urol* 1996; 29: 145–54.

23. Van Kerrebroeck P, Jardin A, Laval KU, van Cangh P, and the ALFORTI Study Group. Efficacy and safety of a new prolonged release formulation of alfuzosin 10mg once daily versus alfuzosin 2.5mg thrice daily and placebo in patients with symptomatic benign prostatic hyperplasia. *Eur Urol* 2000; 37: 306-13.

24. Jardin A, Bensadoun H, Delauche-Cavallier MC, Attali P, BPH-ALF group. Alfuzosin for the treatment of benign prostatic hypertrophy. *Lancet* 1991; 337: 1457–61.

25. McNeill SA, Pallon D, Iain M et al. SR-alfuzosin and trial without catheter following acute urinary retention: a prospective, placebo-controlled trial. *Eur Urol* 1999; 5(Suppl.2): 76–79.

26. Imperato-McGinley J, Guevro L, Gauteri T, Petersen RE. Steroid 5-alpha-reductase deficiency in a man: an inherited form of pseudohermaphroditism. *Science* 1974; 186: 1213–5.

27. Stoner E. The clinical effects of a 5-alpha-reductase inhibitor, finasteride, on benign prostatic hyperplasia. *J Urol* 1992; 147: 1298–302.

28. Gormley QJ, Stoner E, Bruskewitz RC *et al.* The effect of finasteride in men with benign prostatic hyperplasia. *N Engl J Med* 1992; 327: 1185–91.

29. Finasteride Study Group. Finasteride (MK–906) in the treatment of benign prostatic hyperplasia. *Prostate* 1993; 22: 291–9.

30. Tammela TLJ, Konturri MJ. Urodynamic effects of finasteride in the treatment of bladder outlet obstruction due to benign prostatic hyperplasia. *J Urol* 1993; 149: 342–4.

31. Kirby RS, Vale J, Bryan J, Holmes K, Webb JAW. Long-term urodynamic effects of finasteride in benign prostatic hyperplasia: a pilot study. *Eur Urol* 1993; 24: 20–6.

32. Kirby RS, Bryan J, Christmas TJ, Vale J, Eardley I, Webb J. Finasteride in the management of benign prostatic hyperplasia – a urodynamic study. *Br J Urol* 1992; 70: 65–72.

33. Guess HA, Heyse JF, Gormley GJ. The effect of finasteride on prostate specific antigen in men with benign prostatic hyperplasia. *Prostate* 1993; 22: 31–7.

34. McConnell JD, Bruskewitz R, Walsh P *et al.* The effect of finasteride on the risk of acute urinary retention and the need for surgical treatment among men with benign prostatic hyperplasia. *N Engl J Med* 1998; 338: 557–63.

35. Gisleskog PO, Hermann D, Hammarlund-Udenaes M, Karlsson MO. A model for the turnover of dihydrotestosterone in the presence of the irreversible 5-alpha-reductase inhibitors GI198745 and finasteride. *Clin Pharmacol Ther* 1998; 64: 636–47.

36. Sufrin G, Coffey DS. Mechanism of action of a new nonsteroidal antiandrogen: flutamide. *Invest Urol* 1997; 513: 429–34.

37. Caine M, Perlberg S, Gordon R. The treatment of benign prostatic hypertrophy with flutamide (SCH:13521): a placebo-controlled study. *J Urol* 1975; 114: 564–8.

38. Stone NN, Clejan S, Ray P. A double-blind randomized controlled study of the effect of flutamide on benign prostatic hypertrophy: side-effects and hormonal changes. *J Urol* 1989; 141: 307A.

39. Eri LM, Tveter KJ. A prospective placebo-controlled study of the antiandrogen Casodex as treatment for patients with benign prostatic hyperplasia. *J Urol* 1993; 150: 90–4.

40. Peters CA, Walsh PC. The effect of nafarelin acetate, a luteinizing hormone releasing hormone agonist, on benign prostatic hyperplasia. *N Engl J Med* 1987; 317: 599–604.

41. Gingell JC, Knünagen H, Kurth KH *et al.* Placebo-controlled double-blind study to test the efficacy of the aromatase inhibitor atamestane in patients with benign prostatic hyperplasia not requiring operation. *J Urol* 1995; 154: 399–401.

42. Radlmaier A, Eickenberg HU, Fletcher MS *et al.* Estrogen reduction by aromatase inhibition for benign prostatic hyperplasia: results of a double-blind, placebo-controlled, randomized clinical trial using two doses of the aromatase inhibitor atamestane. *Prostate* 1996; 29: 199–208.

43. Berges RR, Windeler J, Trampisch H *et al.* Randomised, placebo-controlled, double-blind clinical trial of beta-sitosterol in patients with benign prostatic hyperplasia. *Lancet* 1995; 345: 1529–32.

44. Champault G, Patel JC, Bonnard AM. A double-blind trial of an extract of the plant *Serenoa repens* in benign prostatic hyperplasia. *Br J Clin Pharmacol* 1984; 18: 461–2.

45. Cukier J, Ducassou J, Le Guillou M *et al.* Permixon® versus placebo. Results of a multicentre study. *Pharmacol Clin* 1985; 4: 15–21.

46. Descotes JL, Rambeaud JJ, Deschaseaux P *et al.* Placebo-controlled evaluation of the efficacy and tolerability of Permixon® in benign prostatic hyperplasia after exclusion of placebo responders. *Clin Drug Invest* 1995; 9: 291–7.

47. Carraro JC, Raynaud JP, Koch G *et al.* Comparison of phytotherapy (Permixon®) with finasteride in the treatment of benign prostatic hyperplasia: a randomized international study of 1089 patients. *Prostate* 1996; 29: 231–40.

48. Stamey TA, Meares EM, Winningham DG. Chronic bacterial prostatitis and the diffusion of drugs into prostatic fluid. *J Urol* 1970; 103: 187–94.

49. Naber KG. Use of quinolones in urinary tract infections and prostatitis. *Rev Infect Dis* 1989; 11(Suppl. 5); S1321–37.

chapter 7

Specialist management of benign prostatic hyperplasia

Although the use of technological intervention and surgery in the treatment of benign prostatic hyperplasia (BPH) falls largely within the domain of the urologist, it is important that family practitioners become acquainted and keep up to date with the options available (Table 7.1). In addition to standard surgical approaches that still consti-

---

Table 7.1 Specialist treatments for benign prostatic hyperplasia

Technological intervention
Prostatic stents (temporary and permanent)
Thermotherapy
Laser ablation
Transurethral needle ablation (TUNA)
Surgery
Open prostatectomy
Transurethral resection of the prostate (TURP)
Transurethral incision of the prostate (TUIP)
Transurethral electrovaporization of the prostate (TVP)

tute the mainstay of treatment for most patients with BPH, new treatment options are being introduced at an unparalleled rate. Increasingly well-informed patients are now asking questions and requesting information about these new treatment methods, not only from urologists but also from their family practitioners.

TECHNOLOGICAL INTERVENTIONAL METHODS

Many attempts, using a variety of new technologies, are being made to develop the 'ideal' interventional treatment for symptomatic BPH; there is a great enthusiasm on the part of urologists to do so. Most of these techniques are aimed at reducing the 'static' element of outflow obstruction – the transition zone volume. All aim to achieve a satisfactory long-term therapeutic effect with fewer complications, lower costs and a shorter hospital stay than required for traditional surgery.

However, as yet none of the new minimally invasive procedures has been judged to replace transurethral resection of the prostate (TURP) when stringent outcome criteria are applied. While the prospects of these techniques in the management of BPH are exciting, it is important that their longer-term clinical value and safety are assessed at an early stage, so that their place in the ever-expanding therapeutic armamentarium of this disease becomes clear.

Prostatic stents

The concept of a metal spiral stent (Fig. 7.1) inserted into the prostatic urethra to relieve symptoms in patients with prostatic enlargement was originally introduced by Fabian in 1980 [1]. The success of the spiral stent in the management of urethral strictures encouraged researchers to investigate its use in the management of prostatic enlargement. Stents have found a small niche for themselves in the management of BPH. They should not be used routinely, because of the rather high incidence of complications – their particular value is

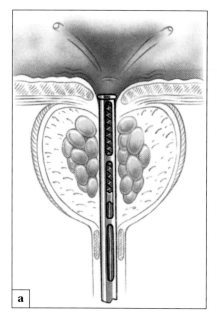 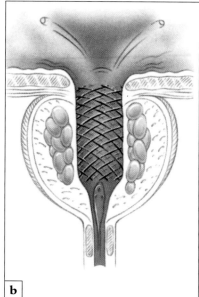

Figure 7.1. Prostatic stent for BPH. (a) Cystoscopic insertion of an expanding 'Urolume' stainless steel prostatic stent. (b) The open stent maintains potency of the prostatic urethra and gradually epithelializes.

in the treatment of acute or chronic urinary retention in patients who are deemed unsuitable for TURP because of severe co-morbidity. Currently available prostatic stents may be either temporary or permanent. In addition, biodegradable stents have been introduced to fulfil a slightly different role.

Temporary stents

Temporary stents, such as the gold-plated Prostakath™, the Nissenkorn™ intraurethral catheter and the more recent thermoexpandable Memokath™, are all associated with complications such as displacement and encrustation. They can be inserted under direct vision cystoscopically or under local anaesthetic using transrectal ultrasound guidance.

When used in patients with acute or chronic urinary retention who are unsuitable for surgery, these minimally invasive procedures are associated with a marked improvement in flow rate. However, associated complications (such as encrustation and migration) and the necessity for the device to be replaced at 6-monthly intervals have limited their role in the treatment of symptomatic BPH [2].

Permanent stents

Permanent stents, such as the Urolume™ [3] and the titanium ASI 'Titan' stents [4] can also be introduced relatively easily and expand to fit the contours of the prostatic urethra. Again, these stents are associated with an excellent short-term relief of obstruction in acute urinary retention (AUR), but only a modest longer-term improvement in flow rate and symptom score in patients with symptomatic BPH who do not present with retention. They are also subject to a number of complications, such as encrustation and hyperplasia of the prostatic urothelium through the holes in the mesh. Patients may also complain of urethral pain and irritation, which currently limits their use to only a very small minority of individuals with outflow obstruction caused by BPH who are unfit for conventional surgery.

Biodegradable stents

Biodegradable stents have been introduced recently to overcome the long period of voiding difficulties that follow certain laser procedures. The use of polymeric composites, such as polyglycolic or polyglactic acid spirals after visual laser ablation of the prostate, has reduced the likelihood of AUR. The stents have ultra high strength, are self-reinforced and are biodegradable; biodegradation occurs in 3–4 weeks with polyglycolic acid and in about 6 months with polyglactic acid [5].

Heat treatment

The idea that local heat cures prostatic disease has been the source of sporadic interest since the 18th century. With the current enthusiasm for new technology, this theory is enjoying something of a renaissance.

Heat treatment for patients with symptomatic BPH is based on the concept that a transrectal probe with rectal protection may be capable of reducing bladder outflow obstruction. Hyperthermia implies an intraprostatic temperature of 41–45°C; this and the higher temperatures within adenomas produced by 'thermotherapy' (45–55°C) have been the focus of many recent studies.

Transrectal and transurethral hyperthermia

Several hyperthermia machines, which use microwave technology to heat the prostate, for example the Prostathermer™ and Primus™ (transrectal), and the Thermex II™ and BSD Prostate™ (transurethral), are all capable of producing an intraprostatic temperature of about 42–44°C (Fig. 7.2). Early reports indicate improvements in peak urinary flow rate and symptom score in about 45% of patients [6]. The group recommended for treatment was, however, fairly restricted, comprising patients with small prostates and only mild-to-moderate symptoms.

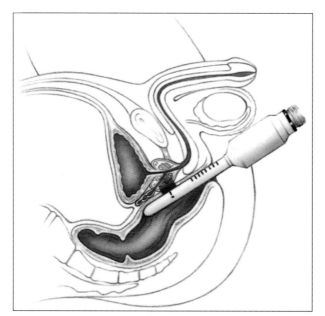

Figure 7.2. Transrectal hyperthermia. The microwave delivery device is passed per rectum and microwave energy directed anteriorly.

Other studies followed, and improvements in both symptom scores and flow rates have been reported using transurethral hyperthermia [7]. However, in a multicentre sham-controlled study of transrectal and transurethral hyperthermia performed in Paris, France, no difference between a sham procedure and treatment with hyperthermia in either subjective or objective criteria was observed, except at 1 year when symptom scores in the treatment group were marginally superior [8]. As a consequence the use of these devices has largely been abandoned.

Thermotherapy

Thermotherapy, or transurethral microwave therapy, is delivered by the Prostatron (Fig. 7.3), which has been extensively evaluated in many centres worldwide. Thermotherapy uses a combination of transurethrally administered heat energy and conductive cooling. The cooling is supposed

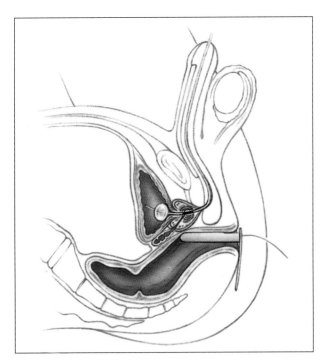

Figure 7.3. Transurethral microwave thermotherapy (TUMT). The 'Prostatron' microwave delivery catheter is passed per urethra and located in the prostatic urethra by inflation of the catheter balloon. Rectal temperature is monitored by means of a device inserted into the rectum.

to prevent urethral damage and pain. The prostatic tissue itself is subjected to a temperature of 45–55°C; these higher temperatures may induce tissue necrosis and possibly induce damage to the intraprostatic nerves and alpha receptors. Several studies have shown significant improvements in symptom scores and peak urinary flow rates using the Prostatron [9].

Recent sham studies [10] suggest that thermotherapy exerts a measurable effect on the prostate, greater than a placebo. A review of many European studies into the use of thermotherapy shows that there is a reasonably long-lasting improvement in peak flow rate of approximately 3 ml/s [11]. These results are achieved using the lower energy package, Prostasoft 2.0. Although no major difference has been found between these results and those achieved with medical treatment of BPH, there is no question that thermotherapy is capable of producing some effect on the prostate. Although the improvements in symptom scores and peak urinary flow rates are not comparable with those of TURP, continued studies with increased energy delivery are justified.

Using higher energy, the Prostasoft 2.5, a higher improvement in peak urinary flow rate can be achieved. Although most of the studies are relatively short-term, it would seem that the average improvement is 5 ml/s at 1 year. The improvement in symptom score is also satisfactory. Balanced against these positive benefits, more significant analgesia and sedation must be used and the requirement for catheterization is increased. Other thermotherapy devices are now available

Laser treatment

Laser technology has been used with increasing enthusiasm in the management of BPH in a number of urological centres (Fig. 7.4). Among its potential advantages are an absence of postoperative bleeding and a minimal in-patient hospital stay.

Although a number of different types of laser energy have been used, the most popular at present is the neodymium:yttrium–aluminium–garnet laser (neodyium:YAG). The laser can be applied either under ultrasound guidance as in transurethral laser incision of the prostate

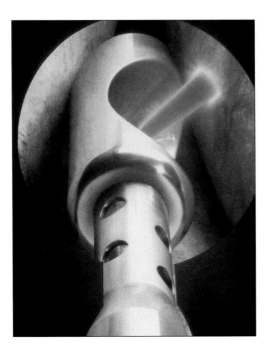

Figure 7.4. Laser ablation of the prostrate. The side-firing delivery probe is inserted through a cystoscope and laser energy applied to the lateral adenoma tissue under vision.

(TULIP), under endoscopic control as in endoscopic laser ablation of the prostate (ELAP), or as interstitial laser ablation (ILAP). Thus, it can be fired at a distance from or directly in contact with prostatic tissue. Many researchers believe laser technology may be one of the standard treatments of the future for prostatic disease because of the lack of bleeding when this technolgy is employed.

Comparisons with TURP have shown that, at least in the short-term, laser prostatectomy results in improvements in symptom score and peak urinary flow rate that are not as good as those of TURP, but are probably better than those of most other technologies. However, the number of certain side-effects is greater than occur with TURP – post-operative infection, length of catheterization, urethral pain and bladder neck stenosis are all more common; postoperative bleeding is, of course, less common with laser technology.

Although the procedure itself is not excessively traumatic for the patient, it still must be performed under some form of anaesthetic. The necessity to stay in hospital is governed by the urologist or patient preference; it is now often offered to the patient as a day-case operation.

The technology is expensive – a laser may cost more than US$100,000 and the laser-deflecting fibres US$500 each. Cost constraints may therefore limit the extensive use of this technology in some units.

Complications

Laser ablation of the prostate occurs at a higher temperature than hyperthermia or thermotherapy, and causes coagulative necrosis of the prostate and subsequent passage of slough. This slough and swelling in response to heat damage is sometimes a problem and, in the immediate postoperative period, most patients have some difficulties in passing urine, as well as some quite persistent perineal and urethral pain. This is managed by a suprapubic or urethral catheter, which must often be left in place for 5 days and sometimes very much longer.

Interstitial laser

The use of lasers described above has been criticized and somewhat limited by side-effects. The visual laser has good results, but further development of laser technology has led to the introduction of the interstitial laser. Laser energy fired in direct contact with prostatic tissue has been further developed into the production of a fibre, which can be introduced into the prostatic tissue itself. Results are similar to those achieved with the other laser techniques, but without the problems caused by sloughing of necrotic tissue. Also, dysuria and voiding difficulties are much less in the short-term.

Latest techniques and developments

New methods of supplying greater degrees of heat to the prostate, and yet preserving the integrity of the surrounding tissues, have been introduced. All of these are at an early stage of development and are undergoing extensive studies to evaluate their effectiveness and safety, and also to assess potential complications.

These techniques are of some interest and may well herald a new dawn not only in the management of BPH, but also in that of prostate cancer.

High-intensity focused ultrasound

High-intensity focused ultrasound causes tissue ablation by inducing high temperatures (90–100°C) in tissues not in contact with, and in fact some distance from, the probe [12]. Thus, by inserting a probe into the rectum high temperatures can be induced in the prostate without damaging the wall of the rectum.

Early clinical studies found that high-intensity focused ultrasound produced symptomatic improvement and an increase in the peak urinary flow rate, although the number of patients treated was relatively small. In a more recent study in a large number of patients over a longer period [13], the peak flow rate had improved at 3 months from a mean of 9 ml/s to 14.4 ml/s, with a corresponding decrease in postvoid residual (PVR) urine and a highly significant improvement in symptom score.

Other independent experimental studies, using a different system but the same principle of high-intensity focused ultrasound, have shown that this technique causes lesions in the prostate (Fig. 7.5) [14]. Early clinical expectations raised by this technology have been dented because, although the concept is an excellent one, the methodology itself is too cumbersome, requires anaesthetic, takes longer than other treatments and yields results that are not sufficiently durable.

Transurethral needle ablation

Transurethral needle ablation (TUNA) using radio waves delivers high temperatures (120°C) to the prostate transurethrally, with no need for an anaesthetic and with minimal disruption to the prostatic urethra (Fig. 7.6). The effects of TUNA are demonstrable both histologically and by magnetic resonance imaging (MRI) and have been corroborated in clinical studies that show marked increases in urinary flow rates from 9 ml/s to as high as 17 ml/s.

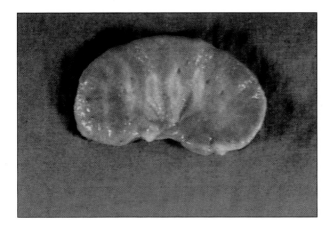

Figure 7.5.
Lesions to the prostate caused by high-intensity focused ultrasound.

A number of trials have been performed with TUNA. A European multicentre open study showed that by 1 year the symptom score had decreased from 22.0 to 7.5, and the peak urinary flow rate had increased from 8.7 to 11.6 ml/s [14]. Although the peak flow improvement was rather less than expected, the symptom score change shows that the technique is valuable. In a US trial comparing TUNA with TURP, the symptom score improvement was similar in both groups, but the improvement in peak urinary flow rate was not as great (6.3 ml/s versus 12.11 ml/s) [15]. In both studies, the complication rate was low, however the device has not become universally popular.

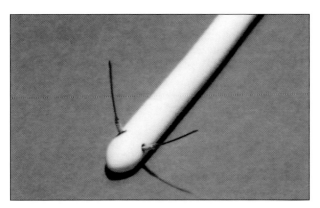

Figure 7.6.
Transurethral needle ablation (TUNA) of the prostate uses radiofrequency antennae to deliver high temperatures to the prostate without anaesthetic.

WATCHFUL WAITING

Is it reasonable to defer treatment in patients with lower urinary tract symptoms by so-called 'watchful waiting'? Under some circumstances, the answer to this is clearly yes. Provided that the patient with mild symptoms has been adequately assessed and has no evidence of malignancy affecting the prostate, a careful period of watchful waiting may well be indicated. Watchful waiting, however, should not be a byword for neglect and it is clearly not an option for those patients who do not wish to tolerate bothersome symptoms any longer or those with absolute indications for surgery (Table 7.2).

SURGICAL OPTIONS

By far the most common procedure is TURP (representing about 95% of prostate operations), although open retropubic prostatectomy may be more appropriate for very large prostates (>100 ml). When the prostate is small and yet is the cause of outflow obstruction and associated perhaps with an obstructive bladder neck, the procedure of choice could well be a transurethral incision of the prostate (TUIP).

Table 7.2 Absolute indications for surgery

- Recurrent episodes of haematuria
- Recurrent attacks of urinary infection
- Acute or chronic retention of urine
- Bladder stones secondary to BPH
- Upper tract dilatation
- Large diverticulum or multiple diverticula

Open prostatectorny

Open prostatectomy is performed through a lower abdominal incision, either midline or transverse suprapubic, and either through the
bladder (transvesical prostatectomy) or through the capsule of the
prostate (Millin's prostatectomy). In both cases, the adenoma is enucleated and a urethral catheter is left to drain the bladder for up to 5 days
postoperatively. The wound usually heals quickly and is not excessively
painful (Fig. 7.7). The procedure is especially suitable for those patients
with very large adenomas (>100 g).

Open prostatectomy is a very effective method of treating benign
prostatic obstruction; symptoms improve markedly and the mean peak
flow usually increases to more than 20 ml/s postoperatively. Furthermore,
the likelihood that patients will require further surgery is lower with open
prostatectomy than with TURP [13]. However, the procedure is more
invasive and requires longer hospitalization than transurethral surgery,
which makes it very much less attractive to patients.

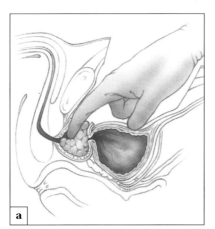
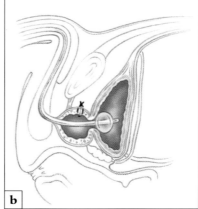

Figure 7.7. Millin's retropubic prostatectomy. (a) An incision is made through
the anterior prostatic capsule and the transition zone adenoma enucleated by
means of finger dissection. (b) The capsule is closed and a Foley catheter is
retained for around 5 days.

Transurethral resection of the prostate

Over the past 50 years TURP is an operation that has become increasingly refined (Fig. 7.8). With the optical systems that are now available, it can be carried out using a visual display on a video screen. The procedure has become relatively easy to perform in experienced hands, but should be undertaken only by surgeons who have been specifically trained and are sufficiently expert in the technique.

The procedure is carried out through a resectoscope with a diathermy loop. Slivers of tissue are excised and then evacuated through the resectoscope sheath. Spinal epidural or light general anaesthetic is usually used and the patient will require a urinary catheter for 36–48 hours postoperatively. Postoperative pain is not usually a problem, symptoms rapidly improve and peak urinary flow rates generally increase to above 18–20 ml/s.

Transurethral incision of the prostate

A simple procedure, TUIP has been practiced since the 19th century (Fig. 7.9). With advances in optic technology, it is now very simple and straightforward. However, TUIP is suitable only for small prostates with a high bladder neck and no middle lobe enlargement. An incision is made from just below the ureteric orifice on one or both sides and carried through the bladder neck to 0.1 cm proximal to the verumontanum. The results are generally excellent, with a postoperative peak flow rate of about 18 ml/s [16]. The incidence of complications is very low, and even retrograde ejaculation occurs in no more than 10% of patients. A proportion of patients, however, do not improve or subsequently relapse, and may subsequently need a TURP.

Transurethral electrovaporization of the prostate

The same technology as is used in TURP and TUIP has now been extended to produce transurethral electrovaporization of the prostate (TVP). The prostate is literally vaporized as a grooved cylinder is passed along its surface (Fig. 7.10). This means that the tissue is removed without the formation of a coagulum, but the haemostasis is excellent. The

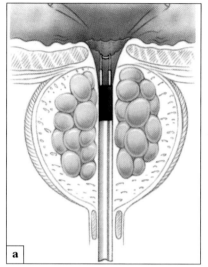

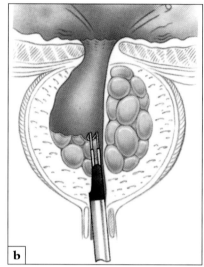

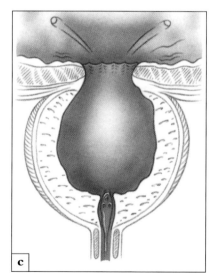

Figure 7.8. Transurethral resection of the prostate (TURP). (a) The median lobe is resected by a resectoscope. (b) Further tissue is then resected until all the transitional adenoma is removed. (c) A 'cavity' persists, which tends to shrink with time.

disadvantage is that no tissue is available for histological examination; the advantages are a decrease in postoperative haemorrhage and a catheterization time of usually no more than 24 hours.

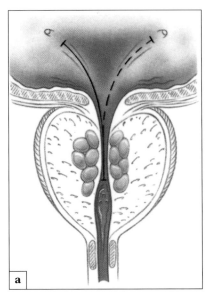 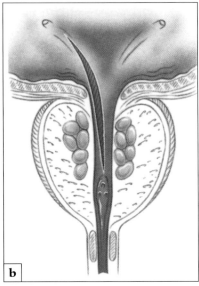

Figure 7.9. Transurethral incision of the prostate (TUIP). An incision is made through the bladder neck area (a) allowing the lateral tissue areas to spring apart (b). Some urologists use a bilateral incision, as shown.

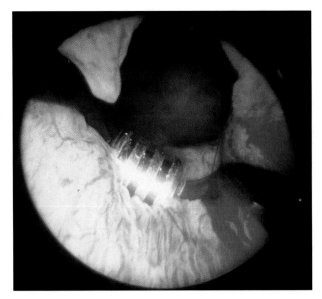

Figure 7.10. Transurethral electrovaporization of the prostate. The grouved cylinder is passed over the prostate under direct vision.

An initial open study showed that TVP was a safe and effective technique. Subsequently, a comparative study between TVP and TURP was made. At 1 year, improvement in symptom score was the same in both groups, while improvement in peak urinary flow rate was comparable (9.7 ml/s for TVP versus 11.3 ml/s with TURP) [18]. Complications were also comparable with both therapies, but haemorrhage was significantly less frequent with TVP. Consequently, the greatest advantage of TVP is a reduced hospital stay. Further multicentre international studies are awaited.

Complications of surgical treatments

Complications of surgical treatments are given in Table 7.3.

Table 7.3 Complications of surgical treatment for benign prostatic hyperplasia

Complications	Transurethral incision of the prostate	Transurethral resection of the prostate	Open prostatectomy
Overall rate	14.0%	16.1%	21.7%
Risk of blood transfusion	2.0%	5–15.0%	30.0%
Incontinence	0.1%	0.8%	0.4%
Erectile dysfunction	12.6%	15.7%	19.0%
Retrograde ejaculation	10.0%	68.0%	72.0%
Need for operative treatment of surgical complications	2.9%	3.3%	4.2%
Likelihood of death within 90 days of surgery	<1.0%	<1.5%	<2.0%

Primary haemorrhage

Primary haemorrhage, which occurs within 24 hours of surgery and is directly related to the surgery itself, is not usually severe. A blood transfusion is necessary in less than 5–15% of patients and hence the policy is now to seldom cross match the patient's blood before TURP.

Clearly, any predisposition to haemorrhage needs to be investigated and appropriate steps taken. Many patients who have had heart valve surgery or myocardial ischaemia and are on warfarin undergo TURP. The warfarin must be stopped 4–5 days preoperatively and cover continued with intravenous heparin. Heparin is stopped 4 hours preoperatively and then reintroduced postoperatively. Patients with a history of ischaemic heart disease may be taking aspirin, which should also be stopped 2 weeks before surgery.

Secondary haemorrhage

Secondary haemorrhage after TURP is often reported to the family practitioner. It generally happens 10–14 days postoperatively and is a relatively common, if minor, occurrence. The patient should be advised to rest in bed, increase his fluid intake and take appropriate antibiotics depending on urine culture and sensitivity reports. Occasionally secondary haemorrhage can be severe; if clot retention supervenes the patient requires urgent hospitalization and catheterization, and occasionally bladder washout to remove the clots.

Urinary incontinence

Urinary incontinence after TURP usually arises from pre-existent detrusor instability with or without sphincter weakness. Urge incontinence is most characteristic, and commonly disappears within a few weeks or months after surgery. Urge incontinence is best treated with anticholinergics, which also, of course, treat the symptoms of frequency and nocturia.

Very occasionally stress incontinence can occur, because of some degree of sphincter damage. Stress incontinence also usually disappears with time, but if after 6 months residual stress incontinence still concerns the patient, the insertion of an artificial urinary sphincter may be occasionally necessary.

Urethral stricture

Urethral stricture is a very disappointing complication of TURP for both patient and surgeon, and can occur in 3–6% of cases [19]. The most frequently affected sites are the external urethral meatus, the bladder neck, the penoscrotal junction and the bulbar urethra. The incidence of strictures after TURP can be minimized by urethrotomy or careful gauging of the size of the urethra with Clutton's sounds, and the use of a resectoscope that fits easily within a well-lubricated urethra. Urethral strictures most commonly present 4–5 months after surgery in patients who have, up to that time, had great relief of their preoperative symptoms; they are usually disappointed at the sudden change in events, when symptoms of outflow obstruction return.

Initial treatment is most commonly direct vision internal urethrotomy. If the stricture is at the meatus, gentle meatal dilatation may be sufficient, Occasionally, optical urethrotomy or reconstructive surgery of the urethra may be required.

Sexual dysfunction

Retrograde ejaculation is the most common sexual dysfunction following prostatectomy (Fig. 7.11). The incidence after TURP and open prostatectomy is about 70%, but only 10% following TUIP. Every patient who undergoes prostatic surgery should, of course, be warned that retrograde ejaculation is likely to occur. Most patients who have been properly informed are not troubled by retrograde ejaculation in the longer term.

Some patients complain of erectile dysfunction after prostatic surgery. While no clear surgical explanation for this has been established, the cavernous nerves and vessels do pass near the apex of the gland. It is worth remembering that in middle-aged and elderly men, pre-existing erectile dysfunction, either psychogenic or physically based, may be present. If the patient wishes, erectile dysfunction can be treated by the oral agent sildenafil (Viagra™), intraurethral prostaglandin E_1 (MUSE™), or intracorporeal injections of prostaglandin E_1 Caverjeck™. The use of implantable penile prostheses and the vacuum pump are also acceptable forms of therapy for some patients.

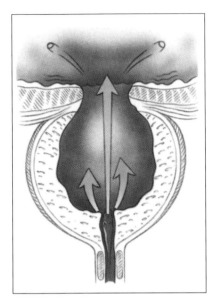

Figure 7.11. Retrograde ejaculation. After TURP, semen passes retrogradely into the bladder at the time of orgasm because of the loss of the bladder neck sphincter mechanism.

Outcome of surgical treatments

While most patients who have had a TURP are perfectly satisfied with the outcome, recent studies have shown that 15–20% have a less than perfect result (Table 7.4) [20]. These findings may reflect a rather nonselective policy for TURP whereby patient selection is generally based on their symptoms, which are nonspecific; sometimes the flow rate may not be absolutely selective either. In addition, patients do not always describe their symptoms or their effect on quality of life as thoroughly to the urologist as they do to their family practitioner. Although recent retrospective studies have shown that the re-operation rate in patients undergoing TURP is higher than in those undergoing open prostatectomy [21], this does not justify an abandonment of the less invasive procedure. The reduction of symptom score and improvement in peak urinary flow rate is greater with either TURP or open prostatectomy than with any other currently available therapy for BPH.

Table 7.4 Outcome of surgical treatment for benign prostatic hyperplasia

Outcome	Transurethral incision of the prostate	Transurethral resection of the prostate	Open prostatectomy
Likelihood of symptom improvement	80%	88%	98%
Reduction in symptom score	73%	85%	79%
Improvement in mean peak flow rate	8–15 ml/s	8–18 ml/s	8–23 ml/s
Likelihood of further treatment within 5 years	8.1%	3.4%	0.4%

Although TURP is a satisfactory and relatively safe method for treating prostatic outflow obstruction, it has been argued that a more careful evaluation of the impact of the symptoms and the presence of obstruction is required before such surgery is undertaken. This is to ensure that only those patients who are both genuinely affected and bothered by true bladder outflow obstruction are subjected to prostatic surgery, which, in turn, should enhance the results obtained (Table 7.4).

Mortality after TURP in the best centres is now less than 0.3% [22], but retrospective studies of cases at all units suggest an overall mortality of about 1.5% [21]. Many patients who undergo prostatectomy have some co-morbid condition that is undoubtedly related to postoperative mortality; patient selection is therefore critical. Serious postoperative sepsis has been virtually eradicated by the use of antibiotic prophylactics.

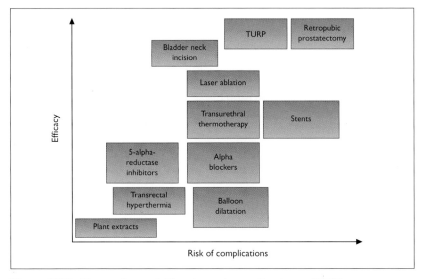

Figure 7.12. Comparison of efficacies and complications of BPH treatments.

Balance-sheet concept and patient-based decisions

As there are insufficient efficacy, safety and long-term outcome data to tailor any particular therapy to each and every individual patient, the 'balance-sheet' concept may be helpful (Fig. 7.12). This involves explaining to the patient that treatment results in both indirect and direct health outcomes. The indirect health outcomes may be of no consequence to the patient's mind (e.g. improvements in flow rate, PVR urine and pressure flow studies), while the direct health outcome, that is improvement in symptoms, is often extremely important. For the patient to make a fully informed decision, the positive effects, the likelihood of successful long-term outcome and the relative incidence of complications for each treatment option must be explained fully.

The importance of providing options so that a patient-based decision can be made cannot be overestimated. Patient counselling may be helped by the recent introduction of interactive videodisks and other digital materials that explain the condition and the treatment options. This may allow a shared decision between patient, family practitioner and urologist based on an understanding of anatomy, pathology and treatment.

CHAPTER SUMMARY

- Acute and chronic retention of urine remain absolute indications for prostate surgery.
- Recurrent urinary tract infections, haematuria due to BPH, bladder stones and upper tract dilatation are also indications for TURP.
- For patients with symptomatic BPH who do not have acute or chronic urinary retention, it is advisable to have a full, informed discussion about the balance of the risks against the benefits of surgery.
- The newer technologies have a role to play in the management of BPH, but their exact clinical utility is still being tested. At present, none has been shown to be superior to TURP, although some have come reasonably close in terms of efficacy. The question of cost-effectiveness still needs to be addressed, as does that of their long-term results in terms of durability of effect.

REFERENCES

1. Fabian KM. Der intraprostatiche 'partielle katheter' (urologiste spirale). *Urologe A* 1980; 23: 229–33.

2. Nordling J, Oversen H, Poulsen AL. Intraprostatic spiral: clinical results in 150 consecutive patients. *J Urol* 1992; 147: 645–7.

3. Chapple CR, Milroy EJG, Rickards D. Permanently implanted urethral stent for prostatic obstruction in the unfit patient. *Br J Urol* 1990; 66: 58–65.

4. Kirby RS, Heard SR, Miller PD *et al.* Use of the ASI titanium stent in the management of bladder outflow obstruction due to benign prostatic hyperplasia. *J Urol* 1992; 148: 1195–7.

5. Talja M, Tammela T, Petas A *et al.* Biodegradable, self-reinforced polyglycolic acid spiral stent in prevention of postoperative urinary retention after visual laser ablation of the prostate-laser prostatectomy. *J Urol* 1995; 154: 2089–92.

6. Zerbib M, Conquy S, Steg A, Martinache PR, Flam T, Fabre B. Localized transrectal hyperthermia in the treatment of obstructive manifestations of prostatic adenoma. Review of the literature and personal experience. *J Urol* 1992; 98: 89–92.

7. Devonec M, Ogden C, Perrin P, Carter S. Clinical response to transurethral microwave thermotherapy is thermal dose-dependent. *Eur Urol* 1993; 23: 267–74.

8. Cockett ATK, Khoury S, Aso Y *et al.*, eds. Other non-medical therapies in the treatment of BPH. *2nd International Consultation on Benign Prostatic Hyperplasia*. Paris: SCI, 1994; 460–91.

9. De La Rosette JJ, Frøehling FM, Debruyne FM. Clinical results with microwave thermotherapy of benign prostatic hyperplasia. *Eur Urol* 1993; 23: 68–71.

10. Ogden CW, Reddy P, Johnson H, Ramsay JWA, Carter S. Sham versus transurethral microwave thermotherapy in patients with symptoms of benign prostatic bladder outflow obstruction. *Lancet* 1993; 341: 14–7.

11. Smith P, Contort P, de la Rosette J *et al.*, eds. Other non-medical therapies. *In: 3rd International Consultation on Benign Prostatic Hyperplasia*. Paris: SCI, 1996: 575–603.

12. Ter Haar G, Rivens I, Chien L, Riddler S. High intensity focused ultrasound for the treatment of rat tumours. *Phys Med Biol* 1991; 36: 1495–501.

13. Madersbarcher S, Kratzik C, Szabo N, Susani M, Vingers L, Marberger M. Tissue ablation in benign prostatic hyperplasia with high intensity focused ultrasound. *Eur Urol* 1993; 23: 39–43.

14. Gelet A, Chapelon JY, Margonari J *et al.* High intensity focussed ultrasound experimentation on human benign prostatic hyperplasia. *Eur Urol* 1993; 23: 44–7.

15. Ramon J, Lynch Th, Eardley I *et al.* Transurethral needle ablation of the prostate for the treatment of benign prostatic hyperplasia: a collaborative multicentre study. *Br J Urol* 1997; 80: 128–35.

16. Bruskewitz R, Issa MM, Roehrborn CG *et al.* A prospective randomized 1-year clinical trial comparing transurethral needle ablation to transurethral resection of the prostate for the treatment of symptomatic benign prostatic hyperplasia. *J Urol* 1998; 159: 1588–93.

17. Orandi A. Transurethral incision of the prostate compared with transurethral resection of the prostate in matching cases. *J Urol* 1987; 138: 810–5.

18. Kaplan SA, Laor E, Fatal M, Te AE. Transurethral resection of the prostate versus transurethral electrovaporisation of the prostate: a blinded, prospective, comparative study with a 1-year follow-up. *J Urol* 1998; 159: 454–8.

19. Lentz MC, Mebust WK, Foret JD, Melchior J. Urethral strictures following transurethral prostatectomy a review of 223 resections. *J Urol* 1977; 117: 194–6.

20. Neal DE, Ramsden PD, Sharples L, Smith A, Powell PH, Styles RA. Outcome of prostatectomy. *BMJ* 1989; 299: 762–7.

21. Roos NP, Wennberg JE, Malenka DJ, Fisher ES, McPherson K, Anderson TF. Mortality and re-operation after open and trans-urethral resection of the prostate for benign prostatic hyperplasia. *N Engl J Med* 1989; 320: 1120–4.

22. Mebust WK, Holtgrewe HL, Cockett ATK, Peters PC. Transurethral prostatectomy: immediate and postoperative complications. A cooperative study of 13 participating institutions evaluating 3885 patients. *J Urol* 1989; 141: 243–8.

chapter 8

Modern management of prostate cancer

Although prostate cancer is the second most common cause of cancer death in men in most developed countries, there is a surprising lack of consensus concerning its management, especially the treatment of earlier localized lesions [1]. The principal reason for this is the difficulty in predicting which lesions will progress to the detriment of the patient, as opposed to those which will remain localized and asymptomatic within the affected individual's natural lifespan. There is also a lack of controlled studies comparing one treatment against another. A number of prospective randomized trials that address these issues are in progress.

The dilemma is highlighted by statistics on prostate cancer from the USA, which calculate that a man living to 75 years of age has a:

- 30% chance of having microfoci of histological prostate cancer
- 10% chance of being diagnosed as suffering from clinical disease
- 2.5% life-time probability of dying from the disease.

Clearly, some men die with prostate cancer rather than as a result of it. However, as the death rate from competing mortalities is now falling and the incidence of clinical prostate disease is increasing, the challenge is to identify and effectively treat the life-threatening lesions in the most effective manner. In this respect, a shared care approach to the earlier diagnosis and more effective follow-up of prostatic disease between family practitioners and urologists is likely to be beneficial to patients.

WHICH LESIONS TO TREAT?

Small-volume microscopic foci

Small-volume microscopic foci of well-differentiated cancer identified at transurethral resection of the prostate (TURP) have little impact on survival. Provided that they are not a harbinger of more significant disease in the peripheral zone, in older patients and those with significant comorbidity these may often be left untreated [2]. This low-volume, microscopic disease, although present in many men, does not seem to be detectable by current methods of screening.

Large lesions

Larger lesions (>0.5 cm^3) are usually more dangerous, as are any histologically less well-differentiated cancers (Gleason grade >3) [3]. These tumours are usually, but not always, associated with:

- a serum prostate-specific antigen (PSA) >4.0 ng/ml
- palpable induration of the prostate (Fig. 8.1)
- an abnormal transrectal ultrasound (TRUS) image and positive biopsies.

The mortality risk associated with such a lesion must always be balanced against the life expectancy of the individual person concerned (i.e. the probability of death from co-morbid conditions,

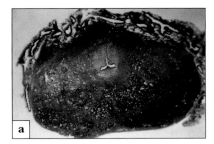 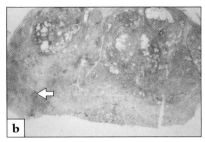

Figure 8.1. (a) Transverse section of a normal prostate. (b) Localized prostate cancer (arrow).

such as cardiovascular disease); clearly, the patient's age, general condition and longevity of his parents are the dominant considerations.

MANAGEMENT OF LOCALIZED PROSTATE CANCERS

Unhappily, in most countries at present, only around 30% of prostate cancers are diagnosed when still confined within the gland. This is probably a reflection of the reluctance of men beyond middle age to consult a doctor about their prostate problems and under utilization of PSA testing. Those cancers that are detected usually need to be evaluated by a urologist and carefully staged on the basis of PSA levels, a bone scan and sometimes computed tomography (CT) or magnetic resonance imaging (MRI). However, even with the latest methods of staging and endocavity technology, up to 30% of apparently localized lesions are found to have spread through the prostatic capsule at the time of surgery. For those lesions that are thought to be localized, several treatment options are available [1].

Watchful waiting

Low-volume lesions
Watchful waiting may be appropriate when the tumour is of low volume and well differentiated (i.e. Gleason grade <4), especially in older patients with other significant co-morbid conditions [4]. However, regular review with repeated PSA determination is important in such cases. Active treatment should be considered, especially in younger men, if there is evidence of local tumour extension or an incremental PSA rise.

Larger-volume lesions
A more aggressive approach may be appropriate for larger-volume lesions (>0.5 cm^3) that contain areas of cancer that are less well-differentiated, in men with a life expectancy of more than 5–10 years.

Radiotherapy

Two radiation modalities are currently in use for patients with local-ized prostate cancer – external beam radiation and brachytherapy.

External beam radiation

External beam radiation therapy using high-energy photons is by far the most commonly used, the most versatile and the most thoroughly evaluated (Fig. 8.2). Treatment usually involves two 2-week courses of radiotherapy on an outpatient basis [5]. The morbidity is acceptably low, with the main side-effects being:

- frequency of micturition due to radiation cystitis
- rectal irritation caused by the inevitable inclusion of the rectum in the treatment field
- subsequent gradual development of erectile dysfunction in 30–50% of cases.

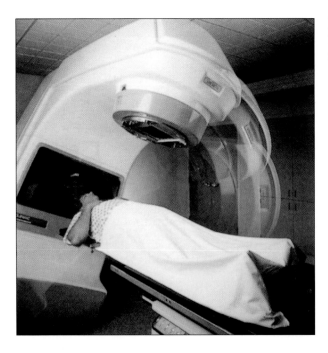

Figure 8.2.
Patient receiving radiotherapy.

The recent introduction of conformal radiotherapy has been reported to reduce the incidence of these side-effects [6].

Although radiotherapy is well tolerated by both younger and older patients, evidence is mounting that many prostatic adenocarcinomas – like colonic adenocarcinomas – are relatively resistant to irradiation. Following a period of PSA decline for some months or years after radiotherapy, many patients experience a PSA rise, which generally heralds a clinical relapse. In addition, several investigators have shown that prostatic biopsies taken 1 year after radiotherapy reveal the presence of viable tumour in 50–60% of patients. Concerns have therefore been raised over the efficacy of radiotherapy in terms of reliable tumour kill. Recently, several studies, including that by Bolla *et al.*, suggested that pretreatment with an luteinizing hormone releasing hormone (LHRH) analogue (so-called neoadjuvant downsizing therapy) and subsequent androgen ablation improves the efficacy of treatment and overall survival of patients [7].

Brachytherapy

Brachytherapy or interstitial implantation using iodine-125, palladium-103 or iridium-192 radioactive sources involves the implantation of radioactive seeds to specific parts of the prostate. A recent development involves the transperineal insertion of the implant needles that contain the radioisotopes under real-time TRUS guidance. This has improved the accuracy of placement and allowed a more uniform distribution of seeds. Using this technique, higher doses of irradiation can be delivered to the prostate than those delivered using external beam radiation.

The technique can be performed on an outpatient basis, using either temporary or permanent implants. Temporary implants contain high-energy sources, such as iridium-192, that are left in the prostate for a specified period of time. Permanent implants contain low-energy sources, such as iodine-125 or palladium-103, that are left in the prostate to decay. However, a recent study comparing brachytherapy, external beam radiation and radical prostatectomy suggests that brachytherapy is only as effective in terms of cancer spread at 5 years as the other two therapies in men with 'low-risk' prostate cancer [8].

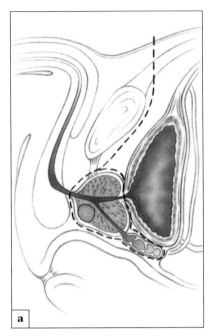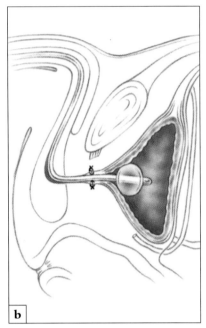

a

b

Figure 8.3. Radical retropubic prostatectomy. (a) The entire prostate and seminal vesicles are excised. (b) The urethra is anastomosed to the bladder over a 22F catheter, which is retained for 2–3 weeks.

Radical prostatectomy

Radical prostatectomy is the most definitive method of clearing the body of malignant prostate cancer cells, provided that the lesion is still confined within the gland (Fig. 8.3; Table 8.1). Agreement is widespread among urologists that patients with localized prostate cancer selected for radical prostatectomy should have a theoretical life expectancy of at least 10 years and no significant co-morbidity.

Complications

Concerns about the morbidity associated with the operation have, however, prevented many urologists from adopting this procedure. The continence and potency-preserving modifications described and popularized by Dr Patrick Walsh have reduced the complication rates

Table 8.1 Comparison of curative therapies for localized prostate cancer

Therapy	Invasiveness	Hospitalization	Complete tumour eradication	Adverse effects
External beam radiotherapy	Nil	Nil	<50%	Rectal irritation Urinary frequency Impotence (30%)
Brachytherapy	Minimal	24 h	50–75%	As above
Radical prostatectomy	Retropubic or perineal dissection	6 days	75%	Impotence (50%) Incontinence (2%)

dramatically; many patients remain potent and incontinence – defined as the need for more than two small pads per day – now occurs in less than 2–5% of cases [9]. Furthermore, the inpatient hospital stay is now only 3–6 days, and the pathological evaluation of the prostate and internal iliac lymph nodes allows precise staging and employment of adjuvant therapy, such as external beam radiotherapy or antiandrogens when appropriate.

Clinical outcome

Provided that the surgical margins are clear, radical prostatectomy reliably reduces serum PSA levels effectively to zero (<0.1 ng/ml), which is very helpful during follow-up. Any detectable level of PSA after radical prostatectomy indicates the presence of residual or recurrent tumour, and further adjunctive therapy, such as radiotherapy or androgen ablation therapy, should be considered.

The number of radical prostatectomies performed annually under Medicare in the USA has steadily risen [10] a trend that is now being followed elsewhere.

MANAGEMENT OF LOCALLY EXTENSIVE PROSTATE CANCER

A proportion of patients with prostate cancer present with extraprostatic extension, but no evidence of more distant metastases. For these cancers, radical surgery is probably inappropriate because of the unacceptably high local and distant recurrence rates.

Radiotherapy
Radiotherapy is usually the preferred treatment option, but evidence suggests that few patients are actually cured by it, although disease progression may be slowed.

Cytoreduction therapy
Recently, cytoreduction therapy has been in vogue. It comprises a 3-month course of hormonal therapy – usually with an LHRH analogue such as goserelin acetate or leuprolide – to achieve tumour shrinkage. Subsequent radiotherapy, or occasionally surgery, may be directed towards a reduced tumour burden. Data from Bolla *et al.* suggest that the combination of androgen ablation with the LHRH analogue goserelin and external beam radiation improves survival [7].

Monotherapy with antiandroandrogens
Previously, many patients with locally-advanced prostate cancer were treated with androgen ablation using either bilateral orchidectomy or LHRH analogues. Recently, it has become apparent that antiandro-

gen monotherapy with bicalutamide (Casodex™) can yield similar results, but avoids the severe impact on sexual function that castration therapy involves [11].

TREATMENT OF METASTASES – ANDROGEN BLOCKADE

Although the proportion of patients with localized disease at the time of diagnosis is now rising, probably as a result of PSA testing, in many countries more than 50% of patients with prostatic cancer still have metastatic disease at the time of presentation. Since the Nobel prize-winning work of Huggins and Hodges on the hormone dependence of prostate cancer in 1941 [12], it has been appreciated that around 70% of such patients respond to therapy directed towards depriving the cancer cells of the androgens necessary for their growth. This may be accomplished by a variety of means, both medical (Table 8.2) and surgical.

Bilateral orchiectomy

Bilateral orchiectomy can be accomplished through a midline scrotal incision under local, regional or light general anaesthetic. The advantages of this procedure are patient compliance, low cost and efficacy in lowering serum testosterone level. The disadvantages are the psychological effect of loosing the testes, surgical morbidity and irreversibility of the hormone ablation. The major side-effects are erectile dysfunction, reported to occur in 50–75% of patients, occasional breast tenderness and hot flushes. For these reasons, most patients choose medical means of achieving castration and must always be given the option. In one survey, 78% of patients selected medical rather than surgical endocrine therapy for their cancer [13].

Luteinizing hormone releasing hormone analogues

Shortly after the decapeptide structure of LHRH had been elucidated, it was realized that modification of three of the component peptides would result in a compound of greatly increased potency. Chronic

Table 8.2 Medical treatment options for advanced prostate cancer.

Type	Agent	Dose	Side-effects
LHRH analogues	Leuprolide	Monthly (soon 3-monthly)	Hot flushes
	Goserelin		Erectile dysfunction
	Buserelin		↓Libido
Nonsteroidal antiandrogens	Flutamide	250 mg q8h	Gynaecomastia
	Nilutamide	300 mg/day	Diarrhoea
	Bicalutamide	150 mg/day	
Progestogenic antiandrogens	Cyproterone acetate	100 mg q8h	Fluid retention Impotence
Oestrogens	Diethylstilboestrol	2–5 mg/day	Impotence Gynaecomastia Cardiovascular toxicity

administration of these agents results in a temporary increase followed by an inhibition of luteinizing hormone (LH) and follicle stimulating hormone (FSH) release from the pituitary, and a subsequent suppression of testosterone secretion similar to that obtained by surgical castration. At present, three forms of LHRH analogue are available:

- leuprolide
- buserelin
- goserelin acetate.

All three are now available as 3-monthly injectable depot formulations. The depot preparations can be administered in a primary care setting, usually by the practice nurse, in conjunction with less frequent follow-up visits to hospital [14].

On initiation of therapy, all LHRH analogues result in a temporary surge of LH production with a resultant increase in testosterone to 140–170% of basal levels. This effect has been described as the 'flare phenomenon', because of the risk of transient stimulation of prostate tumour growth. This may result in an increase in bone pain and enlargement of spinal metastases with a risk of neurological complications, including paraplegia.

For this reason, it is recommended that for the first 4 weeks after starting an LHRH analogue, adjunctive treatment with an antiandrogen, such as bicalutamide 50 mg or flutamide 250 mg q8h, should be employed.

The advent of LHRH antagonist such as abarelix which is currently in phase III trials will avoid the need for antiandrogen cover against tumour flare.

Prognosis

Clinically, medical castration with an LHRH analogue is equally as effective as orchiectomy, providing about a 60–80% objective response rate [15]. The reversibility of LHRH treatment offers patients an acceptable option to identify whether or not their disease is hormone sensitive before making a definitive decision about their treatments.

Antiandrogens

Four antiandrogenic agents have been extensively evaluated clinically for the treatment of metastatic prostate cancer – cyproterone acetate, flutamide, nilutamide and bicalutamide.

Cyproterone acetate

Cyproterone acetate is a steroidal antiandrogen with marked progestational activity; it inhibits LH release from the pituitary, produces castrate levels of testosterone and also competes with testosterone and dihydrotestosterone (DHT) for androgen receptor sites. However, if it is used as monotherapy, there tends to be a gradual increase in testosterone values with chronic usage as a result of gradual loss of pituitary inhibition, so this agent may not be as effective in the long term as diethylstilboestrol (DES) or orchiectomy. There have also been reported cases of liver tumour induction and other forms of liver toxicity.

Cyproterone acetate, in doses as low as 50 mg/day, is also useful in the treatment of the troublesome 'hot flushes' that may result from androgen withdrawal following orchiectomy or LHRH analogue therapy.

Flutamide

Flutamide is a nonsteroidal antiandrogen that has been used as monotherapy for metastatic prostate cancer. It has not, however, received regulatory approval anywhere in the world for this indication and, at present, flutamide should always be used in conjunction with either medical or surgical castration. There are data to suggest that when flutamide is used as monotherapy it leaves around 40% of androgen receptor sites still available for binding by DHT; when combined with castration, however, only 5% of DHT is able to interact with androgen receptors. Flutamide does not lower plasma testosterone levels; indeed, levels may be increased.

Unlike most other agents active against prostate cancer, flutamide when used alone does not usually affect libido and potency. Diarrhoea, however, is not uncommon, and gynaecomastia and breast tenderness also occur, presumably because of increased aromatization of testosterone to oestradiol. These latter effects are not seen when flutamide is combined with an LHRH analogue, such as leuprolide, goserelin or buserelin.

Nilutamide

Nilutamide is another nonsteroidal antiandrogen similar to flutamide. In contrast to cyproterone acetate, nilutamide is devoid of progestational and antigonadotrophic properties. It competes with testosterone and DHT at the androgen receptor, not only at the level of the prostate, but also at the hypothalamopituitary complex (where androgens exert their negative feedback effect). As a result, LH secretion is enhanced and, in the presence of intact testes, testosterone biosynthesis is increased. However, because of the presence of the antiandrogen, the effects of rising testosterone at the receptor level are blunted.

Theoretically, therefore, nilutamide, like flutamide, is not ideal as monotherapy and currently no data support its use in this context. Its main value seems to be in combination with an LHRH analogue. Side-effects of nilutamide include gastrointestinal symptoms, anaemia and disturbances of light–dark adaptation.

Bicalutamide

Bicalutamide (Casodex™) is a nonsteroidal antiandrogen that binds to the androgen receptor in the rat prostate with about 2% of the affinity of DHT, but roughly four times the affinity of flutamide. Phase II clinical trials revealed reasonable efficacy of bicalutamide 50 mg/day when used as monotherapy in patients with metastatic prostate cancer, as judged by both serum acid phosphatase and PSA level decline. The most common side-effects were breast tenderness, gynaecomastia and hot flushes; however, the incidence of hot flushes was lower in those who received bicalutamide (19%) than in those treated by orchiectomy (58%). In humans, bicalutamide does, like flutamide, appear to elevate serum testosterone levels markedly, because of central antagonism of T receptors in the hypothalamopituitary complex, with a consequent increase in LH secretion [16]. This has led to concern about its ability to block androgen receptors completely in the nuclei of androgen-sensitive cells. However, bicalutamide has a long half-life which enables high serum concentrations to be maintained; moreover, in patients treated with bicalutamide, serum testosterone concentrations rarely exceed the normal levels at the androgen receptor that the drug must antagonize.

Bicalutamide 50 mg has proved less effective than castration in two of the three Phase III studies that have been conducted; end points were either time to treatment failure or time to progression [17]. Other studies using dosages of 100, 150 and 600 mg are ongoing. A Phase III study compared bicalutamide 150 mg/day as monotherapy with either the LHRH analogue, goserelin, or orchiectomy. Interim results suggest equivalence between the treatments in patients with locally-advanced disease, but a slight advantage in the LHRH arm in patients with proven bone metastases [11].

Maximal androgen blockade

Although LHRH and orchiectomy produce good initial responses in the majority of patients, these are not usually maintained in the long-term. Androgen-independent cancer cell lines develop and the mean time to progression is only 18–26 months, with a mean overall survival time of 28–36 months. Adrenal androgen secretion may contribute to this poor prognosis. This has lead to the concept of maximal androgen blockade (MAB), in which LHRH therapy or orchiectomy is combined with an antiandrogen.

Impetus towards a more rigorous evaluation of the clinical effect of MAB came from the demonstration that up to 10–15% of intraprostatic DHT remains after medical or surgical castration [18]; moreover, it has been confirmed that adrenal androgens may be responsible for as much as 15–20% of total intraprostatic DHT [19].

In response to these observations, a prospective randomized placebo-controlled trial was established in the USA in 1984. The protocol was simple in its design, and compared leuprolide 1 mg/day subcutaneously, plus placebo with leuprolide 1 mg/day subcutaneously, plus flutamide 250 mg q8h in patients with metastatic cancer of the prostate confirmed on radioisotope bone scan. Overall survival was improved in the group who received flutamide, particularly those with a good performance status and a lesser burden of metastatic disease (Fig. 8.4) [20]. Other studies [21–27] comparing various alternative regimens of total androgen blockade with monotherapy have not always confirmed such unequivocal advantage (Table 8.3).

The first meta-analysis of MAB used data from seven randomized, double-blind studies that compared orchiectomy plus nilutamide with orchiectomy plus placebo in 1056 patients with advanced prostate cancer [28]. The group that received MAB had a significant reduction in disease progression and also a 10% reduction in the risk of death (not significant). The most recent meta-analysis by the Prostate Cancer Trialists' Collaborative Group included 22 trials with a total of 5710 patients [29]. Overall mortality was 56.3% in those who received MAB compared with 58.4% in those who received

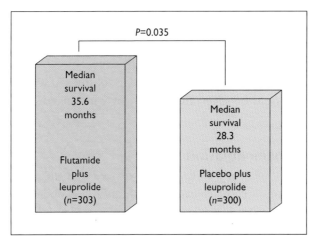

Figure 8.4. Survival is increased in patients with metastatic cancer given combination therapy with leuprolide and flutamide, compared with those given Leuprolide alone [20].

Table 8.3 Summary of studies of maximal androgen blockade.

Study	Agent	Additional progression-free survival (over monotherapy)	Additional overall survival (over monotherapy)
Crawford et al. [20]	Leuprolide plus flutamide	2.6 months*	7.3 months*
Lunglmayr [26]	Goserelin plus flutamide	Nil	Nil
Denis [23]	Goserelin plus flutamide	Significant $p = 0.009$	7 months**
Janknegt [25]	Orchiectomy plus nilutamide	5.9 months*	7.0 months*

*$p<0.05$; **$p<0.04$

medical or surgical castration alone. Five-year survival estimates were 26.2% with MAB and 22.8% with castration alone.

Nonetheless, there is still a role for MAB over conventional monotherapy, at least in fitter patients with smaller volumes of metastases who probably should be given the benefit of what may be the most effective therapy.

Intermittent androgen ablation

Intermittent androgen ablation has been investigated as a means of avoiding the progression of prostate cancer to an androgen-independent state. Endocrine therapy is given intermittently, the logic being that serum testosterone levels return to normal during the periods off treatment. This stimulates atrophic cells and makes them sensitive to the next round of androgen ablation. This approach is still under investigation and is not a recommended form of therapy for prostate cancer.

Other methods of achieving androgen blockade

Diethylstilboestrol

Although inexpensive, DES is associated with significant cardiovascular toxicity at doses of 5 mg/day or 3 mg/day. This toxicity is reduced at a dose of 1 mg/day, but serum testosterone levels are not reliably suppressed into the castrate range [30]. One European study, however, in which patients were randomized to either DES 1 mg/day or bilateral orchiectomy, with or without cyproterone acetate, showed no differences in either survival or cardiovascular thromboembolic events. Also, DES causes troublesome gynaecomastia (Fig. 8.5) and, in most circumstances, is no longer first-line therapy for prostate cancer, but may sometimes be helpful in patients who suffer hormone escape. Because of its known thromboembolic effects it should be used in combination with aspirin.

Finasteride

Finasteride is a 4-azasteroid competitor of 5 alpha-reductase, the enzyme that converts testosterone into DHT within the prostate, and

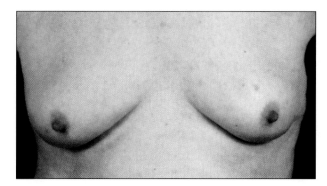

Figure 8.5.
Gynaecomastia as a result of diethylstilboestrol therapy.

is also used as therapy for BPH (see Chapter 6). Several studies have confirmed that finasteride reduces serum DHT by 60–75% while maintaining testosterone levels, and results in significant regression of the benignly enlarged gland [31]. Finasteride has been associated with a marked decline in intraprostatic DHT, but a rise in intraprostatic testosterone levels. Animal studies suggest that finasteride may have activity in prostate cancer [32], and a pilot study in 28 patients with metastatic prostate cancer showed a small reduction in PSA, rather less than that seen after orchiectomy or treatment with an LHRH analogue [33]. It seems likely that androgen receptors in prostate cancer metastases do not demonstrate the selective responsiveness to DHT, as opposed to testosterone, that characterizes both normal prostate and BPH tissue. However, a study of 120 patients randomized to either finasteride or placebo after radical prostatectomy showed an 18-month delay in PSA rise in the drug treatment group [34]. Finasteride in combination with an antiandrogen might also have some efficacy without inducing impotence [35].

Finasteride is a competitive inhibitor of type II 5 alpha reductase, while other newer inhibitors, such as dutasteride, inhibit both type I and type II 5 alpha reductase. A report of the use of epristeride in androgen-responsive cell lines and in R-3327 tumour-bearing rats suggested some potentially useful antitumour activity [36]. The appeal of a 5 alpha-reductase inhibitor in this context is the very favourable toxicity profile compared with the other agents discussed above; virtually the only side-effect seen with finasteride is a 3–5% incidence of impotence, which is usually reversible on discontinuation of the drug.

TIMING OF ENDOCRINE ABLATION FOR METASTATIC PROSTATE CANCER

Traditionally, urologists have favoured deferred administration of hormonal manipulation in patients with prostate cancer – often waiting until symptoms appear before acting to ablate testicular androgens. The rationale for this decision to delay therapy was largely based on a study that showed no difference in average survival rates between patients given hormonal therapy and those in whom hormonal therapy was withheld and placebo given until they became symptomatic [37]. However, recent re-analysis of these data, in which deaths from cardiovascular events in the oestrogen-treated group were excluded and cancer-specific death rates calculated, showed that patients who were treated initially with oestrogen therapy fared better than those treated with placebo [38]. This finding has been corroborated by the recent Medical Research Council trial of immediate versus deferred therapy [39], which showed that overall survival was significantly prolonged in the patients treated early. In support of this approach, laboratory studies have shown that early hormonal therapy does not result in earlier androgen resistance [40]. It is now generally agreed that prompt intervention in patients who present with metastatic disease is beneficial, both in terms of time to progression and overall survival.

MANAGEMENT OF 'HORMONE-ESCAPE' METASTATIC PROSTATE CANCER

Unfortunately, after a period of response to androgen ablation almost all prostate cancers eventually begin to grow again; this is termed 'hormone escape'. Ideally, second-line therapy to obtain a second remission would be used, as in the management of carcinoma of the breast. Unfortunately, no second-line therapy has been confirmed efficacious and safe in this respect, although many new agents, including angiogenesis inhibitors, tyrosine kinase and growth factor inhibitors, are currently being tested in this context. Prednisolone in high doses may also produce a useful symptomatic response, although the mechanism remains unclear.

The most common clinical problem is debilitating bone pain from bone metastases (Fig. 8.6). Local radiotherapy to painful areas may be

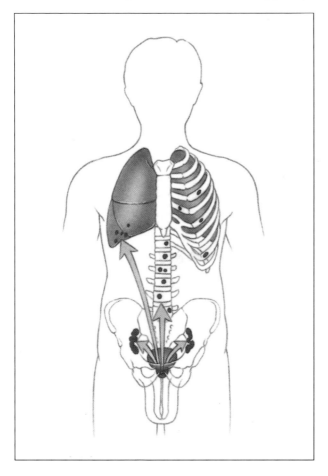

Figure 8.6.
Prostatic cancer commonly spreads to lymph nodes, bones and lungs. These metastases may cause local symptoms

also of value or, if the discomfort and deposits are very diffuse, intravenous strontium-89 [41] may achieve useful palliation.

However, despite all efforts, most patients with hormone-escape prostate cancer deteriorate remorselessly and die within months of the first signs of relapse.

LOOKING AHEAD

The optimal management of prostate cancer now requires care to be shared between the urologist and the family practitioner. The initial treatment strategy should be devised by a specialist on the basis of tissue diagnosis and careful staging. Radiotherapy or prostatectomy are obviously the province of the hospital-based team, but initial diagnosis and follow-up can be the joint responsibility of urologist and family practitioner. Metastatic disease is increasingly managed by monthly or 3-monthly depot injections of LHRH analogues, which may be administered as readily by the family practitioner or practice nurse as by the urologist. There is now evidence to support the early introduction of endocrine therapy at the time of diagnosis rather than waiting for symptoms to develop [39]. The family practitioner may also play a key role in the palliative therapy and terminal care of patients with advanced disease.

The hypothesis that androgen precursors secreted by the adrenal glands may play a role in maintaining prostate cancer growth and the escape of tumour cells from hormone control after ablation of testicular androgens has its advocates. There is some evidence that a subgroup of patients with 'good performance' (i.e. those that are in good general condition) and a reasonably restricted volume of metastatic disease may, in fact, remain in remission longer and have a more prolonged survival if treated by total androgen blockade, as opposed to conventional monotherapy.

In the future, it may be possible to predict, by biochemical or morphometric means, a subgroup of patients in whom total androgen blockade, rather than monotherapy, may offer a definite survival advantage. Newer, more effective first- and second-line curative pharmacotherapies also need to be developed. These challenges may be added to the many others that must be overcome to reduce the morbidity and mortality of this prevalent and insidious disease.

CHAPTER SUMMARY

- Optimal management of prostate cancer may now requires shared care between urologists and family practitioners.
- Microscopic foci of well-differentiated prostate cancer have little impact on survival and often require no treatment, especially in older men or those with significant co-morbidity; by contrast, larger lesions (>0.5 cm^3) and those that are moderately or poorly differentiated carry a poorer prognosis and may warrant more aggressive treatment.
- Curative treatment options for prostate cancer include radical prostatectomy and external beam radiotherapy or brachytherapy. Locally advanced lesions may be treated by prior hormonal manipulation (cytoreduction) followed by external beam radiotherapy.
- Metastatic prostate cancer is usually treated by androgen withdrawal, which has a response rate of 70–80%. Treatment options include bilateral orchiectomy or the use of LHRH analogues. The use of oestrogens is associated with an increased risk of cardiovascular side-effects and gynaecomastia.
- The addition of an antiandrogen (such as flutamide, nilutamide or bicalutamide) to achieve MAB by neutralizing the 5% of residual androgens secreted from the adrenal glands, may possibly increase both the time to disease progression and provide a survival advantage in some patients with good performance status and less advanced metastatic disease, although this is still controversial.

- Current second-line therapies after relapse add little life-expectancy at present, although many new compounds are under investigation.
- Palliative treatment, which often involves the province of the family practitioner, is usually given for bone pain or anaemia. It involves the use of blood transfusions, corticosteroids, local radiotherapy and intravenous strontium-89, but seldom significantly improves survival.

REFERENCES

1. Kirby RS. Treatment options for early prostate cancer. *Urology* 1998; 52: 948–62.

2. Matzkin H, Patel JP, Altwein JE, Soloway MS. Stage T1A carcinoma of the prostate. *Urology* 1994; 43: 11–21.

3. McNeal JE, Bostwick DG, Kindrachuk RA, Redwine EA, Freiha FS, Stamey TA. Patterns of progression in prostate cancer. *Lancet* 1986; i: 60–3.

4. George NJR. Natural history of localized prostate cancer managed by conservative therapy above. *Lancet* 1988; 1: 494–7.

5. Bagshaw MA, Cox RS, Ramback JE. Radiation therapy for localized prostate cancer *Int J Radiol Biol Phys* 1986; 12: 1721–7.

6. Dearnaley DP, Khoo VS, Norman *et al.* Comparison of radiation side-effects of conformal and conventional radiotherapy in prostate cancer: a randomized trial. *Lancet* 1999; 353: 267–72.

7. Bolla M, Gonzalez D, Warde P *et al.* Improved survival in patients with locally advanced prostate cancer treated with radiotherapy and goserelin. *N Engl J Med* 1997; 337: 295–300.

8. D'Amico AV, Whittington R, Malkowicz SB *et al.* Biochemical outcome after radical prostatectomy, external beam radiotherapy or interstitial radiation therapy for clinically localized prostate cancer. *JAMA* 1998; 280: 969–74.

9. Catalona WJ, Bigg SW. Nerve-sparing radical prostatectomy: evaluation of results after 250 patients. *J Urol* 1990; 143: 538–44.

10. Lu-Yao GL, Greenburg ER. Changes in prostate cancer incidence and treatment in the USA. *Lancet* 1994; 343: 251–4.

11. Tyrrell CJ, Denis L, Newling D *et al.* Casodex 10–200 mg daily, used as monotherapy for the treatment of patients with advanced prostrate cancer. An overview of the efficacy, tolerability and pharmacokinetics from three phase-II dose-ranging studies. Casodex Study Group. Eur Urol 1998; 33: 39–53.

12. Huggins C, Hodges CV. Studies of prostatic cancer: I Effect of castration, oestrogen and androgen injections on serum phosphates in metastatic carcinoma of the prostate. *Canc Res* 1941; 1: 293–7.

13. Cassileth BR. Patients' choice of treatment in stage D prostate cancer. *Urology* 1989; 33 (Suppl. 5): 57–61.

14. Debruyne FMJ. Long-term therapy with a depot luteinizing hormone-releasing hormone analogue (Zoladex) in patients with advanced prostatic carcinoma. *J Urol* 1988; 140: 775–7.

15. Kaisary AV, Tyrell CJ, Peeling, Griffiths K. Comparison of LHRH analogue (Zoladex) with orchiectomy in patients with metastatic prostatic carcinoma. *Br J Urol* 1991; 67: 502–8.

16. Kennealey GT, Furr BJA. Use of the non-steroidal antiandrogen Casodex in advanced prostatic cancer. *Urol Clin North America* 1991; 18: 99–110.

17. Iversen P. Update of monotherapy trials with the new antiandrogen, Casodex (ICI 176,334). *Eur Urol* 1994; 26(Suppl.): 5–9.

18. Geller J, De La Vega DJ, Albeit JD. Tissue dihydrotestosterone levels and clinical response to hormone therapy in patients with prostate cancer. *J Clin Endocrinol Metab* 1984; 58: 36–40.

19. Harper ME, Pike A, Peeling WB Griffiths K. Steroids of adrenal origin metabolized by human prostatic tissue both in vivo and in vitro. *J Endocrinol* 1974; 60: 117–25.

20. Crawford ED, Eisenberger MA, McLeod DG *et al.* A controlled trial of leuprolide with and without flutamide in prostatic cancer. *N Engl J Med* 1989; 321: 419–24.

21. Mayer FJ, Crawford ED. Optimal therapy for metastatic prostate cancer. In: Hendry WF, Kirby RS, eds. *Recent Advances in Urology/Andrology.* Edinburgh: Churchill Livingstone, 1994: 159–75.

22. Schellhammer PF, Sharifi R, Block NL *et al.* Clinical benefits of bicalutamide compared with flutamide in combined androgen blockade for patients with advanced prostatic carcinoma: final report of a double-blind, randomized, multicenter trial. Casodex Study Group. *Urology* 1997; 50: 330–6.

23. Denis LJ, Keuppens F, Smith PH, *et al.* Maximal androgen blockade: Final analysis of EORTC phase III trial 30853. EORTC Geniko-Urinary Track Cancer Cooperative Group and the EORTC Data Center. *Eur Urol* 1998; 33: 144–51.

24. Canadian Anandron Study Group. Total androgen ablation in the treatment of metastatic prostate cancer. *Semin Urol* 1990; 8: 159–65.

25. Janknegt RA. International Anandron Study Group: efficacy and tolerance of a total androgen blockade with Anandron and orchidectomy. A double-blind, placebo controlled multicentre study. *J Urol* 1991; 145: 425A.

26. Lungmayr A. The international prostate cancer study group. A multicentre trial comparing the LHRH analogue Zoladex, with Zoladex plus flutamide in the treatment of advanced prostate cancer. *Eur Urol* 1990; 18(Suppl. 3): 28–9.

27. Iversen P, Sucini S, Sylvester R. Zoladex and flutamide versus orchidectomy in the treatment of advanced prostate cancer. A combined analysis of two European studies EORTC and DAPROCA 86. *Cancer* 1990; 66: 1067–73.

28. Bertagna C, DeGiery A, Hucher M *et al.* Efficacy of the combination of nilutamide plus orchiectomy in patients with metastatic prostate cancer. A meta-analysis of seven randomized double blind trials (1056 patients). *Br J Urol* 1994; 73: 396–402.

29. Prostate Cancer Trialists' Collaborative Group. Maximum androgen blockade in advanced prostate cancer. An overview of 22 randomized trials with 3283 deaths in 5710 patients. *Lancet* 1995; 346: 265–9.

30. Shearer RJ, Hendry WF, Sommerville IF. Plasma testosterone, an accurate monitor of hormone treatment in prostate cancer. *Br J Urol* 1973; 45: 668–77.

31. Gormley GJ, Stoner E, Bruskewitz RC *et al.* The effect of finasteride in men with benign prostatic hyperplasia. *N Engl J Med* 1992; 327: 1185–91.

32. Brooks JR, Berman C, Nguyen H *et al.* Effect of castration, DES, flutamide, and the 5-alpha-reductase inhibitor MK906, on the growth of the Dunning rat prostatic carcinoma, R-3327. *Prostate* 1991; 18: 215–7.

33. Presti JC, Fair WC, Andriole G. Multicentre randomised double-blind, placebo controlled study to investigate the effect of finasteride (MK906) on stage D prostate cancer. *J Urol* 1992; 148: 1201–4.

34. Andriole G, Block N, Boake R. Two years of treatment with finasteride after radical prostatectomy. *J Urol* 1994; 151: 435A.

35. Kirby RS, Robertson C, Turkes A *et al.* Finasteride in association with either flutamide or goserelin as combination hormonal therapy in patients with M1 carcinoma of the prostate. Prostate 1999; 40: 105–114.

36. Lamb JC, Levy MA, Johnson RK, Issacs JT. Response of rat and human prostatic tumours to the novel 5-alpha-reductase inhibitor, SK&F 105657. *Prostate* 1992; 21: 15–34.

37. Veterans Administration Cooperative Urological Research Group. Carcinoma of the prostate: treatment comparisons. *J Urol* 1967; 98: 516–9.

38. Sarosdy MF. Do we have a national treatment plan for stage D1 carcinoma of the prostate? *World J Urol* 1990; 8: 27–32.

39. The Medical Research Council Prostate Cancer Working Party Investigators Group. Immediate *vs.* deferred treatment for advanced prostate cancer. Initial results of the Medical Research Council trial. *Br J Urol* 1997; 79: 235–46.

40. Isaacs JT. Timing of androgen ablation therapy and/or chemotherapy in the treatment of prostate cancer. *Prostate* 1984; 5: 1–7.

42. Laing AH, Ackery DM, Bayly RJ *et al.* Strontium-89 chloride for pain palliation in prostatic skeletal malignancy. *Br J Radiol* 1991; 64: 816–22.

chapter 9

Case studies

CASE 1: BLADDER OUTFLOW OBSTRUCTION DUE TO BENIGN PROSTATIC HYPERPLASIA

A 69-year-old man presents with a 2-year history of daytime frequency, nocturia and poor stream. He also has a history of hypertension and is currently being treated with atenolol and a thiazide diuretic. On examination, no abnormal physical signs are found other than a blood pressure of 140/95 mmHg and a benign enlargement of the prostate on digital rectal examination (DRE). How would you proceed?

Family practitioner: Start by taking a careful history, enquiring about nocturia, strength of urinary stream and the degree of bother that the symptoms cause – the so-called 'three questions'. An International Prostate Symptom Score (IPSS) would be helpful. The impact of the symptoms on the patients' quality of life (and on that of his family!) is important. A focused physical examination should be performed including a cardiovascular check and a DRE. An electrolyte and creatinine check should be requested, together with a prostate-specific antigen (PSA) determination. Urine should be tested with a dipstick for haematuria. If available, a bladder ultrasound before and after voiding and a urinary flow rate determination should be requested.

RESULTS

■ Three questions	All positive
■ IPSS	15
■ Degree of bother	Moderate to severe
■ Urea and electrolytes (U&E)	Normal
■ Creatinine	Normal
■ PSA	3.8 ng/ml
■ Dipstick	Negative
■ Bladder ultrasound	Postvoid residual (PVR) volume 180 ml
■ Maximum flow rate	8.4 ml/s

Family practitioner: This patient has moderately severe symptoms of bladder outflow obstruction (BOO) due to benign prostatic hyperplasia (BPH). There is also a history of cardiovascular disease. There is little to suggest a diagnosis of prostate cancer and I would be happy to manage this patient initially with medical therapy, referring him on to a urologist if there was only a modest response to treatment. A repeat IPSS three months after commencement of therapy would help to document objectively the response to treatment. After that I would simply review him annually.

Urologist: This patient is certainly suitable for medical management of his BOO by the family practitioner. A number of considerations, however, need to be borne in mind. Medical therapy could be initiated with either an alpha blocker or a 5 alpha-reductase inhibitor, such as finasteride. If an alpha blocker is chosen, either tamsulosin or alfuzosin could be added safely to the existing antihypertensive regime. Alternatively, doxazosin or terazosin could be substituted for the atenolol and thiazide diuretic. An alpha blocker should produce rapid symptom relief. An alternative is to use finasteride, which should be effective in a patient with an enlarged prostate and a PSA well above 1.6 ng/ml. Finasteride should not only improve symptoms (gradually over a 6-month period), but also reduce the risk of acute urinary retention (AUR) and diminish the chances of surgery becoming necessary.

CASE 2: POSTMICTURITION DRIBBLE

A 56-year-old man presents with postmicturition dribble, but a reportedly normal flow rate. His prostate felt normal on DRE. How would you proceed?

Family practitioner: Patients with this fairly common presentation have little in the way of significant pathology, but are basically seeking reassurance. Referral to a urologist is inappropriate unless the patient requires further reassurance. The answers to the 'three questions' are usually all negative and the IPSS is less than 8. Counsel the patient about postmicturition dribble, informing him that it is a common and benign symptom caused by the pooling of urine in the bulbar urethra. Also, measure creative and PSA to establish a baseline and ask for a midstream urine (MSU) to exclude microscopic haematuria or urinary tract infection (UTI).

Urologist: Postmicturition dribble usually results from pooling of urine in the bulbar urethra after the distal urethral sphincter has closed. Normally, the bulbocavernosus muscles – the ejaculatory muscles – contract around the urethra to expel the last few drops of urine. With time, however, and particularly after any kind of urethral surgery, they function less well and postmicturition dribble occurs. No invasive therapy is indicated. The individual should be advised to exert pressure in the perineum immediately after micturition to empty the bulbar urethra into the pendulous urethra, from which it drains by gravity. Referral is unnecessary in most of these patients.

Occasionally, patients with urethral strictures, or a 'baggy' urethra from previous surgery for stricture disease, may present with these symptoms, in which case a urethrogram may be indicated. Patients with strictures usually admit to a very poor stream and the flow rate is markedly reduced.

CASE 3: ASYMPTOMATIC, CONCERNED PATIENT

A 50-year-old man attends the family practice and requests a prostate health check having read about prostate problems in a newspaper. How would you proceed?

Family practitioner: First, ascertain whether this man has, in fact, any urinary symptoms by asking the 'three questions'. Next ask him to complete the IPSS. It is also advisable to assess his level of knowledge, worries and expectations. Perform a DRE, which would probably be normal in this case, run through some routine laboratory investigations, including serum creatinine and PSA, and send a urine sample for culture and microscopy.

RESULTS

- Three questions   All negative
- IPSS   5
- DRE   Normal
- Serum creatinine   Normal
- PSA   1.6 ng/ml
- MSU   Normal

Family practitioner: All these results are normal. The patient is effectively asymptomatic and he is really looking for reassurance about prostate cancer. With a PSA value of 1.6 ng/ml, advise him that the chances of prostate cancer are extremely low and that no action is necessary, but he should return to the clinic after 1 year for a repeat DRE and PSA determination. Encouraging the adoption of a more healthy lifestyle, including a balanced diet, may be beneficial for the patient.

Urologist: It is worth asking the patient whether or not any first-degree relatives have developed carcinoma of the prostate, particularly at a young age. There is certainly nothing to suggest either outflow obstruction or prostate cancer, and no indication to refer him for ultrasound studies, flowmetry or transrectal ultrasonography (TRUS), but a repeat PSA after 1 year could be considered in a man with these sorts of anxieties. A PSA increment of more than 20% (or >0.75 ng/ml) over 1 year can indicate the development of localized prostate cancer. In a recent study from Seattle, USA, 17% of patients whose PSA levels were originally less than 4 ng/ml, but which rose by more than 20% over 1 year, were found to have prostate cancer when sextant transrectal prostate biopsies were carried out.

CASE 4: FEVER, FREQUENCY AND DYSURIA

A man aged 45 presents with a fever, frequency and dysuria of 10 days' duration. On examination, his prostate is enlarged, has a rather 'boggy' feeling, and is acutely tender on examination. How would you manage this individual?

Family practitioner: This kind of history and physical findings suggests a diagnosis of UTI with acute prostatitis. Send the urine specimen for culture, check his serum PSA and serum creatinine together with a full blood count (FBC) and erythrocyte sedimentation rate, and start this patient on an aminoquinolone antibiotic such as ciproxin. Then arrange to see him when the results of these investigations become be available (about 1 week's time). If there is no response to treatment by then, consider a referral.

RESULTS

- MSU   White blood cell count (WBC) +++, *Escherichia coli* on culture
- Serum creatinine   Normal
- FBC   WBC 15.5×10^6/L
- PSA   40 ng/ml

Family practitioner: These results suggest acute prostatitis. The patient will most likely respond to antibiotics, so plan to keep him on this medication for at least another 3 weeks. Send another MSU at 1 week to see whether the culture at this stage is negative and whether there is any change in the sensitivities of the organism. Allow at least 3 months to lapse before repeating the PSA, which should then have fallen quite steeply. It is also advisable to image the kidneys by ultrasound.

Symptoms of acute bacterial prostatitis
- Fever/malaise
- Pain on ejaculation
- Perineal, low back and rectal pain
- Urinary urgency and frequency
- Nocturia and dysuria
- Bladder neck obstruction of varying degrees.

Urologist: This case certainly is suggestive of a UTI with associated acute prostatitis. The only concern about these patients is that they occasionally develop an intraprostatic abscess and, in such situations, oral antibiotics may not always penetrate the abscess and sterilize the lesion. Occasionally, the patient needs to be hospitalized for intravenous antibiotics and the abscess drained transurethrally. In addition, patients with acute prostatitis can develop quite severe symptoms of BOO and occasionally even develop acute urinary retention (AUR).

An elevated PSA of 40 ng/ml is not at all surprising in a case like this, and indicates the degree of disruption to the prostate caused by the acute infection. As mentioned above, the PSA is expected to drop to normal values within 3 months or so of therapy. If this did not occur, the patient should be referred for TRUS-guided prostatic biopsy to exclude any coincidental malignant process within the prostate.

CASE 5: LOWER URINARY TRACT SYMPTOMS AND A HARD PROSTATIC NODULE

A man aged 62 presents with moderate lower urinary tract symptoms (LUTS) of at least 2 years' duration. On examination, however, his prostate is not enlarged, but has a nodule about 1.5 cm in diameter, which is palpable in the left lobe of the prostate. What are the next steps?

Family practitioner: Clearly, both some degree of BPH and concomitant prostate cancer is suspected in this patient. Check FBC, U&E and creatinine, and send blood for PSA level determination. Refer him urgently, there and then, to a urologist and chase up the PSA results.

RESULTS

- FBC   Normal
- U&E/serum creatinine   Normal
- MSU   Negative
- PSA   12.5 ng/ml

Family practitioner: This PSA result in the absence of much prostatic enlargement and in the presence of a palpable nodule strongly suggests the presence of prostate cancer. In a man of this age, his evaluation by a urologist should be expedited.

Urologist: A man with a PSA of 12.5 ng/ml and a nodule in the prostate has a more than 60% chance of having prostate cancer on biopsy. He needs a TRUS-guided biopsy of the nodule on the left side, as well as sextant biopsies through the rest of the prostate to determine whether or not other concomitant foci of cancer are present.

RESULTS

- Biopsy   Gleason score 2 + 2, well-differentiated cancer in two of the biopsies from the left lobe; all the other biopsies revealed benign tissue

Urologist: These findings suggest the presence of significant-volume cancer in one lobe of the prostate. Provided that the patient has no other significant cardiovascular or respiratory disease, we would consider a magnetic resonance image (MRI) scan of the prostate and pelvic lymph nodes, and definitely perform a bone scan to exclude the presence of either lymphatic metastases in the internal iliac lymph nodes or, more commonly, bone metastases. A recent study found that more than half the patients with a PSA greater than 10 ng/ml had cancer beyond the confines of the prostatic capsule.

RESULTS

- Bone scan   Negative
- MRI scan   No evidence of extraprostatic, seminal vesicle or internal iliac lymph node involvement by tumour

Urologist: The treatment options in this patient are radical radiotherapy versus radical prostatectomy. Unfortunately, no adequately conducted head-to-head randomized prospective studies of these modalities of treatment are available to guide us, but many urologists now believe that radical prostatectomy is more effective than radiotherapy, at least in younger patients with organ-confined lesions. This is because radiotherapy does not reliably bring down the PSA to undetectable levels or render the patient tumour free on repeat transrectal biopsy at 1 year in more than 50% of cases. A new treatment modality, brachytherapy to the prostate, is currently being evaluated in the USA, but at this stage must be considered investigational.

A patient in his early 60s with a biopsy-proven carcinomatous prostatic nodule (stage T2a or T2b) should probably have a radical prostatectomy or radical radiotherapy if his bone scan is negative. With surgery, the patient is usually discharged from hospital within 4–7 days, with the urethral catheter *in situ*. He is readmitted to the day ward 2 weeks later for removal of the catheter. Some initial frequency and urgency may be present, but this usually clears up quickly. There may also be some early stress incontinence, but in an otherwise healthy 62-year-old man this should not persist. In older patients, stress incontinence may be present for a somewhat longer period of time, but urinary continence is regained eventually in most patients: less than 3% have permanent leakage. Erectile dysfunction may occur despite the use of a nerve-sparing technique; however, most patients respond to self-injection therapy with prostaglandin E$_1$ and some to sildenafil (Viagra™).

This individual did undergo a radical retropubic prostatectomy, which confirmed that the tumour (containing areas of Gleason score 6 adenocarcinoma) was confined to the left lobe of the prostate; this extended up to, but did not obviously involve, the capsule on the left-hand side. Postoperatively, he did well with no stress incontinence after removal of his catheter. His PSA remains below 0.1 ng/ml at the time of writing but he does suffer from erectile dysfunction.

CASE 6: LOWER URINARY TRACT SYMPTOMS, LOWER BACK PAIN

A 65-year-old man presents with a history of lower back pain with concomitant LUTS. Clinical examination reveals some tenderness of the lumbar spine with restricted movements, and DRE reveals an irregular stony hard prostate. What are the next steps in this situation?

Family practitioner: The clear suspicion here is prostatic cancer with skeletal metastases, so proceed with the initial investigations of a FBC, U&E and serum creatinine together with a PSA determination, radiographs of the lumbar spine and a request for a bone scan. Urgently refer the patient to a urologist.

RESULTS

- FBC   Normal
- U&E   Normal
- Serum creatinine   Normal
- PSA   249 ng/ml
- Radiography   Lumbar spine – evidence of sclerotic deposits in the lumbar spine and pelvis
- Bone scan   Positive for multiple metastases
- TRUS   Hypoechoic areas suggestive of prostate cancer and capsular distortion
- Biopsy   Positive for adenocarcinoma Gleason score 4 + 4

Urologist: This is a classic case of a patient with metastatic prostate carcinoma. Unfortunately, more than 50% of patients who currently present with prostate cancer are found to have either locally extensive or metastatic disease, and curative therapy in such cases is not possible. A patient like this would most likely be best treated with hormone therapy and at present the evidence suggests that the combination of either orchiectomy or the use of a luteinizing hormone releasing hormone (LHRH) analogue plus an antiandrogen, usually flutamide 250 mg q8h or bicalutamide 50 mg q24h. The rationale behind the addition of these antiandrogens to either orchiectomy or the LHRH analogue is to block the effect of the 5% or so of androgens secreted by the adrenal glands, which are still circulating. In such circumstances, about 70% of men are expected to respond with a rapid PSA decline, with a rapid improvement in the patient's symptoms. Hormone manipulation, as described above, gives the most effective pain relief and, in many cases, no further analgesia is required. Unfortunately, a long-term response to treatment cannot be guaranteed: about half the patients suffer PSA relapse within 18–24 months and there is a 50% or so mortality within 36 months.

Follow-up and palliative control of metastatic bone pain is very much in the province of the family practitioner ideally in consultation and collaboration with the urologist and the palliative care team.

CASE 7: BOTHERSOME LUTS AND RELUCTANCE TO UNDERGO SURGERY

A 56-year-old man presents with bothersome urinary symptoms. On examination his prostate gland is enlarged, but feels benign, and his PSA level is at the upper limit of normal at 3.9 ng/ml. The patient has recently remarried, has read about medical therapy in the press and is keen to avoid any kind of surgical intervention. How do you manage this problem?

Family practitioner: This patient seems to have obstructive BPH, so his answers to the 'three questions' will probably be positive and his IPSS can be expected to be above normal. Check that his prostate is only benignly enlarged on DRE and that his urinalysis, creatinine and PSA are within normal limits. Before starting medical therapy, if possible, obtain a flow rate and ultrasound determination of PVR. At present, most creatine ultrasound and flow rate measurements are obtained through the local hospital, the report coming back to the practice. Some practices, however, are installing their own equipment for these investigations.

RESULTS

- IPSS   14
- PSA   3.9 ng/ml
- Maximum flow rate   9.6 ml/s
- PVR   120 ml

Family practitioner: These results are consistent with BOO due to BPH, and medical treatment is appropriate. His PSA is, however, at the upper limit of normal, so it is advisable to discuss this with a urologist over the telephone. The current choice of medical treatments is between the 5 alpha-reductase inhibitor finasteride or one of the newer longer-acting alpha blockers. As the symptom relief afforded by the 5 alpha-reductase inhibitor can take several months to become evident, a combination of both finasteride and an alpha blocker, such as doxazosin or terazosin, starting off at 2 mg/day and gradually titrating to 5 mg/day over a month, could be used. Tamsulosin or altuzosian could also be employed.

Before patients are started on alpha blockers, they should be warned that about 10% of patients experience drowsiness or mild dizziness, and occasionally nasal stuffiness. Finasteride has a very good side-effect profile and reduces the incidence of AUR and the need for surgery by about 50%, although about 3–5% of patients experience reduced libido and occasionally impotence. A new agent, dutasteride may be available shortly if it proves effective in trials.

Follow-up of patients on medical therapy for BPH is important, and they should be assessed at 3-monthly intervals. After 1 year of therapy, repeat the ultrasound and flow rate measurements, and request a new PSA, which should have fallen to around 50% of the pretreatment value as a result of the effect of finasteride on the PSA-elaborating epithelium. If the subjective and objective responses are good, continue therapy indefinitely.

Urologist: It is certainly unnecessary these days for every patient of this type to be referred to a urologist, but it does mean that the family practitioner has to move up the learning curve in terms of the interpretation of IPSS flow rate measurements, PVR determinations and PSA results. Discussion with a urologist is useful if any doubt exists. As has been mentioned above, the use of finasteride is expected to result in a significant reduction of PSA; the median decline in those patients treated in the phase III double-blind studies was 50%. Those patients with carcinoma of the prostate who were inadvertently included in the phase III studies showed a much smaller decline in PSA and, in most cases, after an initial decline, the PSA value started to rise. These findings indicate that those patients in whom the PSA level does not fall significantly, and especially those in whom a PSA rise is seen in spite of therapy compliance with finasteride 5 mg/day, should be referred for TRUS and prostatic biopsy to exclude prostate cancer. Patients need to be educated about the continued need for compliance, as the beneficial effects of finasteride take time to develop. At present, however, compliance does not seem usually to be a problem.

CASE 8: ACUTE URINARY RETENTION AND SEXUAL CONCERNS

A 58-year-old man who has a much younger wife, but who has been known to have prostatic symptoms for some time, as well as occasional UTIs, and who has been managed by watchful waiting because of worries about sexual dysfunction resulting from surgery, recently presented to the local Accident and Emergency Department with AUR. A catheter was passed and he was told that surgery is likely to be necessary, but will almost inevitably induce retrograde ejaculation. He was discharged home with his catheter *in situ*, and subsequently presents to the family practitioner to discuss the possibilities of alternatives to surgery in the management of his urinary retention.

Family practitioner: Refer this patient to a urologist. Medical treatment with 5 alpha-reductase inhibitors or alpha blockers is seldom of any great value once outflow obstruction has reached the stage of AUR. While he is in the office, however, perform a DRE, and take blood for a PSA and creatinine determination and a specimen of urine from the catheter for microscopy and culture.

RESULTS

- DRE   Marked BPH
- Microscopy   Red blood cell count (RBC)+++
- Urine culture   Negative
- PSA   9.3 ng/ml (elevated in AUR)

Urologist: In patients who present with AUR and who fail trial without catheter, the only recognized management at present is transurethral resection of the prostate (TURP) or open prostatectomy. The results of this form of treatment are excellent, with the virtual assurance for the patient of a satisfactory outcome. We are seeing quite a few patients now who have AUR, but are determined to avoid TURP and request alternative forms of therapy. Unfortunately, none of the new nonsurgical forms of intervention can reliably re-establish voiding in these cases. A trial without catheter after starting alpha blocker therapy is usually unsuccessful. Thermotherapy using the Prostatron device also has an unacceptably high failure rate, and prostatic stents are used only in a highly select group of patients, particularly those with severe, concurrent illness.

Other than a standard TURP, the only treatment that could be considered at present is a laser-assisted prostatectomy. Before undertaking any form of endoscopic laser ablation of the prostate, however, the patient must understand clearly that this is a new technique that should, at this stage, be regarded as investigational. With the use of a side-firing laser fibre, we have managed to re-establish voiding in patients such as this who are very keen to avoid the side-effect of retrograde ejaculation. However, it must be said that retrograde ejaculation can occur even after a laser prostatectomy because of laser damage to the bladder neck mechanism, and the catheter may need to stay *in situ* for some weeks after therapy. In addition, some patients complain of marked dysuria for many weeks after this procedure. Interstitial laser therapy is another possibility for this case.

CASE 9: LOWER URINARY TRACT SYMPTOMS AND CARDIOVASCULAR CO-MORBIDITY

A 66-year-old retired man presents complaining of increased frequency of micturition by night and day, and of a long-standing reduction in the force of his urinary stream. He is known to have angina and has some degree of cardiac failure, which resulted in treatment with a diuretic in the form of frusemide 40 mg/day as well as an ACE inhibitor and sublingual nitrates. He has been aware that his urinary symptoms have deteriorated since the diuretic was started, and he therefore avoids his medication in the morning if he plans to go outside the house. On examination, he is not in cardiac failure and the bladder is impalpable. On rectal examination, the prostate was asymmetrically enlarged, but smooth, and did not feel hard. His PSA was 10.2 ng/ml. How should this problem be dealt with?

Family practitioner: This case is consistent with a patient with BPH; the raised PSA probably reflects the considerable benign enlargement of the gland. Referral, however, should be considered for two reasons:

■ to confirm that the raised PSA is a result of benign rather than malignant disease;

■ because the patient's prostatic symptoms interfere with the efficiency of therapy for his cardiac failure.

Other information that would be helpful in the referral letter would be:

- IPSS
- creatinine and electrolytes
- MSU result
- uroflow, if available in the practice

    Medical therapy with finasteride is a possibility if the results of transrectal biopsy confirm the diagnosis of BPH, but the patient should be warned that the onset of symptom relief may take some months.

Urologist: Yes, even if the prostate felt benign on DRE, as the PSA is over 10 ng/ml, TRUS and a biopsy should be undertaken to confirm a diagnosis of BPH before deciding on management. Assuming that the biopsies all showed BPH, this patient is probably best managed by TURP for rapid and complete relief of outflow obstruction. That is, of course, providing the cardiologists were happy that the anaesthetic necessary for TURP – epidural or light general – did not pose an undue risk due to his mild heart failure and history of angina.

CASE 10: NOCTURIA AND NORMAL FLOW

A 74-year-old man presents mainly with symptoms of nocturia. According to him, his urinary stream is quite normal, but he does admit to drinking quite large quantities of tea and beer in the evenings. What advice would you give him?

Family practitioner: Ask the 'three questions' and, in this case, positive answers on both nocturia and bothersome factor can be expected. His IPSS score would probably be above 8, and DRE might reveal some mild benign enlargement of the prostate. However, the point to remember here is that prostate size does not correlate with the presence or absence of obstruction. As the patient reports a normal urinary stream, his symptoms may well be based on a high fluid intake in the evenings, which produce nocturnal polyuria not associated with outflow obstruction. However, patients do not always have a good perception of the normality of their stream, so obtain a PSA determination, a bladder ultrasound and an objective measurement of flow rate of this man.

RESULTS

- IPSS   14
- Creatinine   Normal
- Blood sugar   Normal
- PSA   3.7 ng/ml
- Maximum flow rate   16.3 ml/s
- PVR volume   30 ml

Family practitioner: These results are reassuring; the prostate appears to be benign, and there is little to suggest significant BOO. This patient might do quite well with simple counselling about reducing fluid intake in the evening. Polyuria in elderly patients may be unrelated to outflow obstruction and does not always indicate prostatic troubles. Careful examination of his cardiac and respiratory systems is therefore necessary, in addition to an MSU, U&E, creatinine and urine analysis for glycosuria.

Urologist: This patient complains of nocturia, but does not have any restriction of voiding. In addition, his flow rate is normal both subjectively and objectively, and his PVR is very low. There is nothing here to suggest that he is severely obstructed. The purists might suggest that he should have a full urodynamic assessment to exclude obstruction, but this may be unnecessary invasive by many urologists. Nocturia can be an extremely 'bothersome' symptom, but it may be caused by many conditions other than BPH. Particularly if nocturia is an isolated symptom, cardiac, renal and hepatic causes should be ruled out.

This patient's symptoms of nocturia are largely self-inflicted as a result of excessive drinking in the evening; stopping this habit should be sufficient. If the patient still complains of symptoms and his flow rate is quite normal, there are two lines of therapy that one might employ:

- Firstly, an anticholinergic agent, such as oxybutynin or detrusitol could be prescribed to try to inhibit unstable detrusor contractions, although this is not always effective in such patients.
- The second and more reliable option is to use an antidiuretic hormone analogue, such as 1-deamino-8-D-arginine vasopressin (DDAVP), which very effectively reduces nocturia and can be administered in tablet form or by intranasal spray. Some patients with urinary frequency occasionally take this treatment during the day in situations when urinary frequency might be socially embarrassing.

CASE 11: PERINEAL DISCOMFORT, DYSURIA AND MALAISE

A 43-year-old man presents with a long-standing history of perineal discomfort associated with intermittent dysuria and a feeling of general malaise. On examination his prostate feels rather indurated, and is markedly tender on palpation bilaterally, but it is not enlarged.

Family practitioner: This history fits a diagnosis of chronic prostatitis and, really the question is whether it is bacterial or abacterial. Undertake a DRE and ask for a urine sample, both before the examination and after, to see whether massaging prostatic fluid into the urethra results in a positive culture of expressed prostatic secretions. Also check the

PSA level. These patients are usually excessively anxious and sometimes do need referring on for specialist investigations, particularly TRUS with colour Doppler imaging.

RESULTS

- MSU — Negative
- Prostate massage specimen — WBC+++
- Culture — Negative
- Maximum flow rate — 15.5 ml/s
- PSA — 0.8 ng/ml
- TRUS — Diffuse hypervascularity of the peripheral zone with abnormal engorgement of the periprostatic veins

Urologist: The criteria for diagnosing chronic prostatitis have already been described in detail. Without prostatic massage and analysis of prostatic secretions, it is a rather difficult condition to diagnose. It can be confused with several ill-defined maladies, such as prostatodynia, which present in a similar manner. Reassurance is important, which may require that the full panoply of investigations be performed. In the absence of bacteria on prostatic massage, antibiotics play only a placebo role and do not have a specific therapeutic function. The use of many compounds for this symptom complex have been studied only in open, non-randomized studies, which do not fulfil statistical evaluation criteria. Microwave thermotherapy or prostatic massage is also probably of little more value than placebo in this condition. Non-steroidal anti-inflammatory analgesics, such as ibuprofen and diclofenac, either orally or as a suppository, may be effective.

It has recently been suggested that the use of an alpha blocker to relax the bladder neck and improve the flow rate of these patients can be useful, but there are no controlled data to confirm this; indeed, no therapy is very effective. The symptoms tend to wax and wane. If pain in the perineum is the predominant symptom, it sometimes helps to refer patients to an expert in chronic pelvic pain. It is also worth rechecking the cultures with a formal lower tract localization test (i.e. massage of the prostate to obtain secretions and collection of divided specimens of urine) to be certain there is no infection within the prostate.

CASE 12: ASYMPTOMATIC, POSITIVE FAMILY HISTORY OF PROSTATE CANCER

A middle-aged man who is asymptomatic, but has a family history of prostate cancer, has noted the recent publicity surrounding this disease and presents asking for a prostate check-up. On examination, his prostate feels of normal size with no areas of induration, but his PSA level is 6.3 ng/ml. How would you deal with this situation?

Family practitioner: This is an increasingly common scenario. The two warning signs in this case are the family history of prostate cancer and elevated PSA. Ask how old the patient's relative was when he developed prostate cancer, and how close a relative he was. The PSA is only mildly elevated, but in a middle-aged man with an apparently normal prostate this could indicate the presence of a tumour. In view of his PSA and family history, this patient should be referred to a urologist for TRUS and biopsy.

RESULTS

- TRUS   Revealed an abnormal hypoechoic area in the left transition zone with hypervascularity on colour Doppler imaging. Biopsy confirmed the presence of an adenocarcinoma of the prostate, Gleason score 2 + 3.

Urologist: Cases with biopsy-proved adenocarcinoma of the prostate now present earlier in many countries because of:

- increased public awareness
- the availability of PSA determinations
- the enhanced ability to biopsy the prostate using TRUS.

A patient with a positive family history of prostate cancer is at more than twice the normal risk of developing prostate cancer, and should be screened carefully. This is an absolute indication for referral to a urologist, who should perform a DRE and PSA, and if any doubt exists as to the interpretation of the results, a TRUS-guided prostate biopsy. This should, in the event of a negative survey, be repeated on a yearly basis. The finding of a PSA of 6.3 ng/ml further increases the index of suspicion and a sextant prostatic biopsy under TRUS control should be undertaken. If the biopsies are positive, the urologist should discuss with the patient the treatment options of radical prostatectomy or radical radiotherapy with or without prior hormonal downsizing with an LHRH analogue.

CASE 13 : ADENOCARCINOMA REVEALED BY TRANSURETHRAL RESECTION OF THE PROSTATE

A 70-year-old man recently presented in the Accident and Emergency Department with AUR and subsequently underwent TURP. Histology revealed BPH in most chippings, but several chips show the presence of well-differentiated adenocarcinoma of the prostate (Gleason score 2 + 2). The patient returns to discuss these results with his family practitioner.

Family practitioner: Explain to the patient the process of TURP and how chippings are sent for pathological analysis. Tell him that the presence of adenocarcinoma of the prostate in two chippings may or may not be significant, but further analysis may be necessary by a urologist. Refer him to the urologist who performed the original surgery.

Urologist: In patients over 70 years of age, we would probably elect for external beam irradiation with careful PSA follow-up. If the conservative option of observation only was adopted in this patient's case, we would suggest 3-monthly PSA determinations, together with a TRUS and biopsy of the residual peripheral zone tissue at 3–6 months after TURP to exclude significant volume residual prostate cancer.

If the PSA increased by more than 20% over 1 year (or more than 0.75 ng/ml in absolute terms), or transrectal biopsies revealed the presence of residual cancer in the younger, fitter patient, more active therapy would be considered. This is defined as a T1a cancer of the prostate. Some studies show that in a healthy patient with a reasonable life expectancy of more than 10 years, definitive treatment by radical prostatectomy or external beam radiotherapy should be suggested. However, TURP is not a satisfactory method of diagnosing prostatic cancer. Many studies have shown that even in this situation a more extensive and more significant peripheral zone cancer can be missed, because TURP removes only the transition zone cancers. The more significant cancers occur in the peripheral zone, and these may be present in association with transition zone cancers.

CASE 14: TRANSURETHRAL RESECTION OF THE PROSTATE AND SEXUAL CONCERNS

A man aged 62 years has seen the urologist and was told that he needs a TURP. He asked his family practitioner what sexual problems could arise from this procedure.

Family practitioner: Patient awareness has increased considerably over the past few years and more time needs to be set aside to discuss the sequelae of surgical procedures more fully. Postoperative sexual problems may cause patients and their partners considerable anxiety – matters that they often find difficult to discuss.

Prostatectomy, whether performed via the transurethral route or retropubic route, interferes with the bladder neck and results in failure of occlusion at the time of ejaculation. This causes retrograde ejaculation and therefore the patient is usually rendered sterile. There is often anxiety about the possible effects of retrograde ejaculation and the patient needs to be reassured that this is not harmful. It may be helpful to explain that, although sterility is universal, erectile problems are a rare complication of prostatectomy. This procedure is normally performed in an age group in which sexual activity is already decreasing and any surgical procedure or major illness may cause impotence.

In the case of TURP, erectile dysfunction may occasionally be caused by the heat generated in the region of the prostatic capsule as a result of resection and coagulation using diathermy. This generation of heat may damage the prostatic nerve plexus through which the corpora cavernosa and corpus spongiosum derive their nerve supply. However, erectile dysfunction occurs in less than 10–16% of patients who undergo this procedure.

Urologist: Erectile dysfunction is a strongly age-related disorder, and many cases that occur after TURP are probably incidental and not the result of surgery. A number of effective forms of treatment are now available for men with this problem. Oral therapy with sildenafil (Viagra™) is now first-line therapy. Intracavernous or intraurethral pharmacotherapy with prostaglandin E_1 is often effective, but it carries a small but significant risk of inducing priapism. Vacuum devices and inflatable penile prostheses are two further treatment options that should be discussed.

CASE 15: TRANSURETHRAL RESECTION OF THE PROSTATE AND COMPLICATION CONCERNS

A man aged 60 years presents to his family practitioner for advice having heard stories from some of his friends about complications of TURP and asks whether he can have the operation performed abdominally to avoid the pain and bleeding he has been told about.

Family practitioner: Advise this patient that retropubic or transvesical prostatectomy has largely been replaced over the past 40 years with endoscopic resection, and now over 95% of prostatic surgery is carried out endoscopically through a resectoscope. These instruments have improved considerably over the years and even very large benign glands can be dealt with in this manner.

The advantages of TURP over open prostatectomy are considerable. It can be carried out under a spinal or epidural anaesthetic, there is no abdominal incision to cause complications with breathing or mobilization and the hospital stay is much shorter. If the gland is extremely large and the risk of blood loss is considerable, or if there is an associated bladder stone or diverticulum that requires treatment, then the retropubic approach may be more appropriate.

In general, prostatectomy by the transurethral route significantly reduces the incidence of postoperative complications. Early mobility reduces the risk of respiratory and thromboembolic complications, and only a small percentage of patients now require postoperative transfusion.

With early discharge from hospital, family practitioners may see bleeding from the prostatic cavity in the early postoperative period, and obstruction by blood clot may require bladder wash-outs and possibly recatheterization. Urinary infection may cause troublesome postoperative dysuria and frequency, but these symptoms respond rapidly to antibiotics.

A rare, but serious, complication in the early postoperative period is the transurethral resection syndrome, which results from absorption of irrigating fluid into the circulation. The fluid overload may produce pulmonary oedema and the glycine, which is metabolized to ammonia, may cause confusion and even transient reversible, blindness.

There may, of course, be the need for a further operation, and estimates vary from 10–20% over a 10-year period. It may be necessary because of recurrent obstructive symptoms caused by further adenomatous deterioration in urine flow or urethral stricture caused by endoscopy. The incidence of urethral stricture is probably only 1–5%.

Finally, it is important to inform patients that TURP does not preclude the development of prostate cancer in the residual prostatic tissue at a later date.

CASE 16: COMPLEMENTARY MEDICINE ENQUIRIES

A man aged 58 years attends the surgery. He is anxious to avoid prostate surgery and is not willing to try medical treatments. He asks your advice about what alternative and complementary medicines are available for his prostatic symptoms.

Family practitioner: As BPH is a variable condition and the severity of the symptoms may fluctuate from week to week, the efficacy of complementary medicine is difficult to evaluate. However, some common-sense advice may be offered to this patient. A healthy diet and lifestyle should be encouraged, with little or no alcohol or tobacco. The diet should contain foods that are high in fibre, low in cholesterol and saturated fats, and include plenty of fresh fruit and vegetables. Constipation should be avoided, and it is probably best to avoid spicy foods, coffee and strong tea, as these substances can increase bladder irritability.

Homeopathy and plant extracts are widely used in Europe, treatments that are claimed to improve prostatic symptoms by influencing both the size of the gland and the state of muscle tone at the bladder neck. It is also asserted that the irritability of the obstructed bladder can be improved, but there are almost no placebo-controlled data to support this.

Medicines commonly available include extracts derived from stinging nettle root, golden rod flowers and the fruit of the saw palmetto. Such treatments have been marketed in Europe, particularly in France, Italy and West Germany, and the pills are available without prescription in most pharmacies in France.

Remedies that contain zinc have been advocated over the past few years, but although zinc is found in high concentrations in the prostate gland in the seminal fluid, the function of this mineral is poorly understood. It has not been shown that the addition of an oral zinc supplement prevents or treats any form of prostate disease or condition.

In all probability most plant extracts are merely an expensive way of administering placebo. Before trying any of these remedies, the patient should certainly be advised to seek medical advice and have any necessary examinations and investigations.

CASE 17: VERY ELDERLY PATIENT WITH SEVERE LOWER URINARY TRACT SYMPTOMS

A 91-year-old man who is mentally alert but physically frail presents with severe lower urinary tract symptoms. He gets up six times in the night and has a very poor urinary flow. What would you advise?

Family practitioner: Very elderly patients, usually with severe symptoms, inevitably have some age-related co-morbidity and are often disturbed by anything that disrupts their normal routine. Carry out a full physical examination, including a DRE. Measurement of PSA is not always necessary because the result does not affect management, but a creatinine and urinalysis are important. Providing the bladder is impalpable and creatinine is normal, consider medical therapy with either an alpha blocker using careful dose titration, or a 5 alpha-reductase inhibitor. Monitor the patient closely with IPSS and, if possible, flow rate determinations to evaluate symptom response.

RESULTS

- MSU   Negative
- Creatinine   Normal
- PSA   Not requested
- Maximum flow rate   8.5 ml/s
- Electrocardiogram   Severe ischaemia
- IPSS   27

Urologist: Very elderly patients usually tolerate hospitalization and general anaesthetic poorly. Although this man is extremely symptomatic and probably severely obstructed, there is a good case for medical management here. However, if chronic or AUR develop, an interventional procedure may be necessary. An occasional alternative to a TURP might be the use of an intraprostatic stent, which could be inserted under local anaesthetic. Stents have been shown to relieve obstruction effectively, but their long-term safety and efficacy is still uncertain.

CASE 18: PROSTATIC INTRAEPITHELIAL NEOPLASIA

A 61-year-old businessman whose father died of prostate cancer is concerned about his own prostate health. He has no urinary symptoms and is otherwise healthy.

Family practitioner: Patients such as these need reassurance. Given the family history I would perform an IPSS, a DRE and request a PSA and creatinine determination. A urinalysis would also helpful.

RESULTS

- IPSS   8
- DRE   Unremarkable
- PSA   4.2 ng/ml
- Creatinine   Normal

In the light of the raised PSA I would refer this man on for specialist assessment and probably biopsy.

Urologist: This man is concerned about the possibility of harbouring, like his father, a prostatic adenocarcinoma. A repeat PSA, with a ratio of free to total PSA, should be asked for and a TRUS-guided biopsy of the prostate organized under antibiotic cover. Careful follow-up is mandatory. A repeat PSA and further prostatic biopsies should be considered. Several series have reported around a 50% probability of a positive result on repeat biopsy in such circumstances. Preventive therapy with vitamin E and selenium has a logic, but there are no studies to confirm efficacy. Finasteride is being tested as a chemopreventive agent in the 5-year randomized study, but no data about its effects in this respect are yet available.

CASE 19: PROSTATE-SPECIFIC ANTIGEN RISE AFTER RADICAL RETROPUBIC PROSTATECTOMY

A 52-year-old banker who had previously undergone a radical prostatectomy for clinically localized prostate cancer attended his family practitioner's surgery and requested a PSA determination. Previous PSA readings after surgery had been below 0.1 ng/ml. This latest PSA value came back at 0.6 ng/ml.

Family practitioner: Follow-up after radical prostatectomy is best managed jointly by the family practitioner and urologist. A PSA that starts to rise is generally an indication of tumour recurrence and an urgent referral is indicated back to the urologist.

Urologist: A PSA rise after radical prostatectomy worries the patient, the family practitioner and the urologist alike. After radical prostatectomy, if the operation has been successful the PSA should remain undetectable (< 0.1 ng/ml). A rise, even to as little as 0.6 ng/ml, usually indicates recurrence and is a cue for further investigations. A TRUS-guided biopsy of the anastomotic area may confirm local recurrence. Alternatively, a bone scan may suggest the development of bone metastases. Often, however, both investigations are negative, in which case a period of watchful waiting, simply monitoring the PSA, is probably the best course of action. Biopsy proof of local recurrence may indicate a course of radiotherapy to the pelvis. If bone deposits become apparent, androgen ablation (usually with an LHRH analogue) should be considered. With either approach a reasonably prolonged response may be anticipated, but unfortunately subsequent relapse usually occurs.

CASE 20: HORMONE ESCAPED PROSTATE CANCER

A 67-year-old accountant presents with a PSA of 17 ng/ml in spite of continuing therapy with an LHRH analogue and an antiandrogen. He had been diagnosed as suffering from metastatic prostate cancer 2 years previously, when his initial PSA was 550 ng/ml.

Family practitioner: This patient would have been jointly managed by the family practitioner and the urologist for the previous 48 months. The initial response to therapy with an LHRH analogue plus an antiandrogen is dramatic, with a rapid PSA decline. The subsequent PSA rise is suggestive of the development of androgen independence and an indication for urgent referral for specialist advice.

Urologist: The management of androgen independent prostate cancer is difficult and sadly seldom very effective. Some manoeuvres are worthwhile, however, including stopping the antiandrogen component of the maximum androgen blockade, because withdrawal of antiandrogens sometimes results in a temporary PSA reduction. Other options include treatment with diethylstilboestrol and aspirin, referral to an oncologist for chemotherapy with mitozantrone or paclitaxel (Taxol), or other experimental approaches such as immunotherapy. Sadly, none of these prove very effective in the longer term and palliative measures, including treatment with corticosteroids and local radiotherapy to relieve local symptoms of bone pain, often prove necessary.

chapter 10

Frequently asked questions

WHAT AND WHERE IS THE PROSTATE?

The normal prostate is a walnut-sized gland that lies at the base of the bladder and surrounds the urethra. Within the gland, secretory cells release prostatic or seminal fluid, which liquefies semen after ejaculation. In benign prostatic hyperplasia (BPH), a progressive enlargement of the gland to the size of a tangerine can occur. The resultant urethral obstruction gives rise to the symptoms of BPH, which are now often referred to as lower urinary tact symptoms (LUTS).

WHAT ARE THE SYMPTOMS OF PROSTATITIS?

Acute prostatitis can present with dysuria, frequency and nocturia, with associated lower back pain. Depending on how severe the attack is, the patient may have pyrexia and sometimes rigors. Chronic prostatitis, on the other hand, presents in a much more low-grade form. The patient may have perineal pain, which sometimes radiates to the penis. This pain is often quite severe, and the condition can be quite difficult to diagnose and eradicate. Diagnosis is made in the recommended way from culture of expressed prostatic excretions.

WHAT ARE THE SYMPTOMS OF BENIGN PROSTATIC HYPERPLASIA?

The symptoms are either 'obstructive' or 'irritative'. Examples of the former are hesitancy, intermittency, terminal dribbling, weak stream and a feeling of incomplete voiding. The 'irritative' symptoms are most commonly frequency, nocturia, urgency and dysuria.

ARE THERE MANY PEOPLE WITH MY PROBLEM (BENIGN PROSTATIC HYPERPLASIA OR PROSTATITIS)?

In older men, BPH is an extraordinarily common disease. Up to 10% of the adult male population experience the bothersome symptoms of BPH. The prevalence increases with age, and up to half of men over 75 years of age require treatment. Although less is known about prostatitis, the prevalence is likely to be almost as high.

ARE THERE TWO FORMS OF PROSTATITIS; ONE THAT RESPONDS TO ANTIBIOTICS, AND ONE THAT DOES NOT?

The causes of prostatitis are not fully understood. When the symptoms are associated with obvious infection, antibiotics are commonly used. When there is no associated infection the rationale for the use of antimicrobial agents is less obvious. Thus, clinical practice identifies two discrete subpopulations, but in both situations the permanent eradication of symptoms may be difficult.

DOES BENIGN PROSTATIC HYPERPLASIA LEAD TO CANCER?

The incidence of both BPH and cancer increases with age. However, it is generally accepted that BPH and prostate cancer are separate diseases with distinct aetiologies.

ARE THERE ANY INTERNET SITES THAT CAN OFFER ME ADVICE AND SUPPORT?

There are a number of very good internet sites providing information about prostatic diseases. They are now too numerous to list. Simply search on the word prostate. You can enter these with anonymity, ask specific questions or look at their frequently asked questions. These sites also contain important links to other sources of information. Happy browsing!

CAN A DOCTOR DIAGNOSE WHETHER I HAVE CANCER OR BENIGN PROSTATIC HYPERPLASIA FROM A DIGITAL RECTAL EXAMINATION?

A digital rectal examination (DRE) is part of the evaluation for BPH, and serves as an approximate index of the size and characteristics of the prostate. Coupled with symptom evaluation, it is considered to be a reasonably reliable determinant of BPH. On its own, it is not sufficiently accurate to serve as a screening test for prostatic cancer.

I AM 50 YEARS OLD. SHOULD I HAVE MY PROSTATE-SPECIFIC ANTIGEN CHECKED REGULARLY?

Measurement of prostate-specific antigen (PSA) when used in conjunction with a DRE enhances prostate cancer detection. Certainly several groups, particularly in the USA, advocate routine measurement of PSA in men aged 50 years or more. However, an issue is that although biopsy is advocated at high PSA levels and no action at an agreed lower level (<4.0 ng/ml), a substantial component of the adult population have intermediate levels and only one out of five turn out to have cancer.

WHY ISN'T PROSTATE-SPECIFIC ANTIGEN MEASURED ROUTINELY IN THE UK?

In fact, if the family practitioner, or more commonly the urologist, has any reason to suspect from other evaluations that prostate cancer may be a possibility, PSA is routinely measured. Routine screening does not take place, however. The rationale is that, as yet, there is no proof from randomized controlled trials that PSA testing and the early diagnosis of prostate cancer reduces the mortality resulting from this disease.

WHAT IS PROSTATE-SPECIFIC ANTIGEN AND WHAT DO THE VALUES MEAN?

PSA is a glycoprotein released by the prostate epithelial cells in proportion to the rate of growth. As prostate cancer is an epithelial-based malignancy, PSA has been used as an early stage index of carcinoma. Although it is commonly used (particularly in the USA), it is not perfect and cannot always reliably differentiate between benign and malignant disease. Values less than 4 ng/ml demand no action and those greater than 10 ng/ml carry a 60% probability of cancer. However, a large component of the population fall in the range 4–10 ng/ml, but only one in five turn out to have carcinoma.

IF MY PROSTATE-SPECIFIC ANTIGEN DROPS, DOES THAT MEAN THAT I AM CURED?

There is no absolute correlation between drop in PSA and 'cure'. Such changes in PSA levels can occur spontaneously or as a result of drug use, e.g. finasteride treatment for BPH. The assessment of cure by the urologist is based on other parameters. In general, though, the lower the PSA after any form of therapy, the better the prognosis for the patient.

MY DOCTOR SAYS I NEED A BIOPSY. WHAT WILL THIS SHOW?

A biopsy is only part of the evaluation for prostatic disease. It may suggest that the specialist is unsure that you have BPH or that there is a possibility of prostatic carcinoma. The procedure involves the removal of 6–8 small portions of prostatic tissue (sometimes under anaesthetic), which is then evaluated by a pathologist and makes a more precise diagnosis possible.

WHAT IS A GLEASON SCORE?

A Gleason score is one of the scoring systems the pathologist uses to assess the stage of any cancer tissue proliferation in biopsies. It is a shorthand that enables the pathologist and urologist to communicate and decide on the most appropriate treatment programme. The range of Gleason score is from 2 to 10. The higher the score, the more aggressive the prostate cancer tends to be.

MY UROLOGIST WANTS TO MEASURE MY UROFLOW. HOW WILL THIS HELP DIAGNOSIS?

Some of the symptoms of BPH may not arise from prostatic growth and subsequent urethral obstruction. In particular, the irritative symptoms (urge and frequency) can arise from changes in the bladder itself. Urodynamic evaluations can help the physician decide whether treatment should be directed towards the prostate, bladder or both.

I HAVE BEEN TOLD THAT I HAVE TO HAVE DRUG THERAPY FOR MY BENIGN PROSTATIC HYPERPLASIA. WHAT ARE THE LIKELY SIDE-EFFECTS?

The most commonly used group of drugs in the treatment of BPH are the alpha blockers (doxazosin, terazosin, alfuzosin and tamsulosin). Up to 20% of patients may feel lethargic and dizzy, with a stuffy nose. In general, most people tolerate these side-effects. As consequence of its mechanism of action, finasteride may cause loss of libido or erectile dysfunction in up to 3–5% of patients who receive it. These side-effects usually wear off if the patient stops taking the medication.

WHAT DECIDES WHETHER I HAVE DRUGS, RADIOTHERAPY OR SURGERY FOR MY PROSTATE CANCER?

If prostate cancer is diagnosed at an early stage, when it is confined to the gland, the patient is usually offered either radical prostatectomy or some form of radiotherapy, either external beam or brachytherapy. Such therapies are potentially curative. If the disease has already spread outside the prostate gland, to bone or some other organ, drug therapy, such as a luteinizing hormone releasing hormone (LHRH) analogue, an antiandrogen or a combination of both, is offered to keep the disease in check rather than to eradicate it completely.

WILL SURGERY INVOLVE REMOVING ALL OF MY PROSTATE?

For BPH, the surgery that is usually offered to the patient is that of transurethral resection of the prostate (TURP). This is performed through the urethra using a resectoscope. The central obstructing part of the gland is removed, leaving the outer rim of the prostate behind; it is similar to the concept of removing the fruit of an orange, and leaving the skin of the orange behind. The operation of radical prostatectomy, which is performed for the removal of localized prostate cancer, does involve the complete removal of the prostate gland and the seminal vesicles.

WILL SURGERY MAKE ME IMPOTENT?

The incidence of impotence, or erectile dysfunction, after TURP is very low, probably somewhere in the region of 10%. However, it depends very much on the age of the patient at the time of surgery as to how commonly erectile dysfunction occurs. For example, if a patient in his early 60s who has been sexually active undergoes surgery, it is unlikely that he will have problems with erections after the operation. On the other hand, if a patient has had waning sexuality prior to surgery, it may well be that he will experience problems. In the case of radical prosta-tectomy, the incidence of erectile dysfunction is somewhat greater than this, probably 60–70%, but some patients recover function over time.

WHAT IS A NERVE-SPARING PROSTATECTOMY?

A nerve-sparing prostatectomy is a type of radical prostatectomy that has been developed by Dr Patrick Walsh of Baltimore. In this an anatom-ical approach is taken to the dissection of the prostate, preserving the nerves to the erectile tissue that pass in the region of the prostate towards the penis. If these nerves are preserved, potency is likely to be spared, while at the same time the entire cancer is removed. If it is felt that the cancer on one particular side extends towards the capsule of the prostate, the neurovascular bundle on that side can be sacrificed while preserving that on the other side. Once again, the results of surgery depend upon the patient's preoperative sexual activity and his age.

IF I BECOME IMPOTENT AFTER SURGERY, WILL SILDENAFIL (VIAGRA™) WORK?

Clinical trials have shown that roughly 50% of men who become impotent after radical prostatectomy respond to sildenafil.

I'M ON TESTOSTERONE INTRAMUSCULAR HORMONE REPLACEMENT THERAPY. CAN THIS RESULT IN ME HAVING BENIGN PROSTATIC HYPERPLASIA OR CANCER?

Although both BPH and prostate cancer are androgen (testosterone) dependent, no evidence indicates that administration of testosterone in this way increases the risk of development. However, careful checks of PSA values are advisable for patients on this therapy.

IS IT POSSIBLE TO CONTROL BENIGN PROSTATIC HYPERPLASIA WITHOUT DRUGS? IF SO WHAT ADJUSTMENTS TO MY LIFESTYLE CAN I MAKE?

Symptoms of BPH can wax and wane naturally and certainly mild symptoms are often 'treated' by watchful waiting. You can control some of the symptoms by reducing fluid intake at night, reducing caffeine intake in general (from not just coffee, but also tea and carbonated drinks), reducing alcohol intake and by stress management.

WHAT IS SAW PALMETTO? DO PLANT EXTRACTS WORK IN BENIGN PROSTATIC HYPERPLASIA?

Saw palmetto is prepared from the fruit of the plant *Serenoa repens*. It is available in over 60 different forms from chemists without prescription. Although no controlled clinical trials have been conducted, some patients experience modest benefit. It is estimated that sales of saw palmetto worldwide are in excess of $1 billion per annum.

MY FAMILY PRACTITIONER WANTS TO PUT ME ON AN ALPHA BLOCKER. DOES IT MATTER WHICH ONE I TAKE?

As a class, all alpha blockers (doxazosin, terazosin, alfuzosin and tamsulosin) produce much the same degree of symptom relief at much the same speed of onset (1 week). It would appear that the level of side effects of existing agents is similar with up to 20% of patients experiencing dizziness and fatigue. However, there is some evidence that the use of newer 'uroselective' drugs such as alfuzosin and tamsulosin can reduce side effect severity and incidence. The incidence of abnormal ejaculation with tamsulosin is also significant. As 40% of BPH patients are hypertensive (a diastolic BP >90 mm/Hg), alpha blockers (such as doxazosin or terazosin) that lower blood pressure may be preferred. It has been argued that tamsulosin or alfuzosin may be better in normotensive patients.

WHAT SIDE EFFECTS CAN I EXPECT FROM MY ALPHA BLOCKER?

It should be remembered that all alpha blockers have some degree of cardiovascular activity; there is a possibility of hypotensive effects on taking the first few doses. All alpha blockers cause some degree of fatigue or lethargy, and can cause dizziness and nasal congestion.

Tamsulosin, uniquely, has a relatively high incidence of retrograde ejaculation associated with its use, but this is not often very troublesome to patients.

WHAT SIDE-EFFECTS AM I LIKELY TO HAVE WITH FINASTERIDE (PROSCAR™)?

The major side-effects of finasteride relate to changes in sexual function. Approximately 4% of patients may experience lowered libido, impotence and/or reduced ejaculate volume. However, the major reason for dissatisfaction is because of the relatively long time required before the drug benefits are observed (6–12 months).

TO TREAT MY BENIGN PROSTATIC HYPERPLASIA, WILL I HAVE TO TAKE A DRUG FOR THE REST OF MY LIFE?

Although there is evidence that the symptoms wax and wane, generally alpha blockers may have to be taken for life, as in the case of hypertension. It has been suggested that finasteride will shrink the gland to an extent that the drug is no longer be required. However, there is no clinical data to support the hypothesis. It should be noted that a small proportion of patients who are medically managed will progress to surgery.

I DON'T WANT TO BECOME IMPOTENT. WHAT BENIGN PROSTATIC HYPERPLASIA DRUG IS BEST FOR ME?

Impotence is associated with the use of finasteride in 3–5% of patients, but is much rarer with alpha blockers. However, tamsulosin may cause retrograde ejaculation.

I HAVE TO HAVE TREATMENT WITH RADIOACTIVE SEEDS. DOES THIS MEAN I AM LIKELY TO BECOME RADIOACTIVE?

This procedure, known as brachytherapy, involves surgical introduction of discretely positioned particles that emit radioactivity. Traditionally, this was achieved by a radioactive beam that could damage surrounding tissue. The seeds emit high-energy particles, but have a short half life (i.e. don't last long). Thus there is little possibility of becoming radioactive.

Index

A

Abarelix, 155
Abdominal examination, 66
Abrams–Griffiths nomogram, 77
Activities of daily living and BPH
    symptoms, 14
Adenocarcinoma, TURP revealing, 194–5
Adenoma
  open prostatectomy, 131
  transurethral resection, 133
Adherence, cell, 54
α-Adrenoceptor blockers, *see* Alpha
    blockers
Africa
  BPH occurrence, 15–16
  prostate cancer occurrence, 18
African descent, North and South
    Americans
  BPH occurrence, 16
  prostate cancer occurrence, 18–20
Age
  in BPH
    acute urinary retention incidence and,
    28, 29
    LUTS occurrence and, 13
  PSA cut-off values and, 73–4
Alcohol and BPH, 16–17
Alfuzosin, 102–4
  FAQs, 210, 213
Alpha-1-antichymotrypsin binding to
    PSA, 72
Alpha blockers in BPH, 95, 97–104, 213–14
  adverse effects, 97, 99, 101, 102, 103, 210,
    213–14
  alpha-1-selective, 99–104
  case study, 184, 185
  FAQs, 210, 213–14, 214, 215

mode of action, 98–9
Alpha-2-macroglobulin binding to PSA, 72
5-Alpha-reductase, 105
  increased activity, in BPH, 48
  reduced activity in Japanese men, 20
5-Alpha-reductase inhibitors
  in BPH, 95, 106–8
  case study, 184
  in cancer, 160–2
  side-effects, 107, 162
  FAQs, 214
Alternative medicine, *see* Complementary
    medicine
America, *see* USA
American dwarf palm, *see* Serenoa repens
Amplifying cells, 50
Androgen(s)
  in BPH pathogenesis, 45, 45–8, 104
  tumour insensitivity to, *see*
      Hormone-escape prostate cancer
Androgen suppression/ablation/blockade,
      see also specific (types of) agents/methods
  in BPH, 96, 104–9
    mode of action, 104–5
  in cancer, 153–63
    intermittent, 160
    in locally extensive disease, 152–3
    maximal, 158–60
    in metastatic disease, 153–62
    radiotherapy and LHRH analogue
      combined with, 149, 152
Angiogenesis, 54
Antiandrogens, *see also specific agents*
  BPH, 108–9
  cancer, 152–3, 154, 155–7
    in advanced disease, 154, 155, 155–7,
      158, 159, 182, 203
    case study, 182, 203

D

E

F

Abbreviations: BOO, bladder outflow obstruction; BPH, benign prostatic hyperplasia; FAQs, frequently asked questions; FP, family practitioner; IPSS, International Prostate Symptom Score; LHRH, Luteinising hormone-releasing hormone analogues; LUTS, lower urinary tract symptoms; QoL, quality of life; SPI, Symptom Problem Index; TURP, transurethral resection of prostate.

The Shared Care Series from ISIS

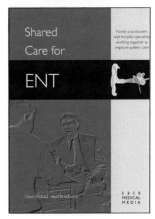

Shared Care for ENT
Chris Milford and Aled Rowlands
ISBN 1-899066-69-1
Paperback, 195 pages

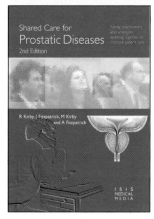

Shared Care for Prostatic Diseases
2nd Edition
Roger Kirby, John Fitzpatrick, Michael Kirby and Andrew Fitzpatrick
ISBN 1-901865-60-6
Paperback, 160 pages

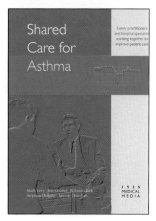

Shared Care for Asthma
Mark Levy, Jon Couriel, Roland Clark, Stephen Holgate and Anoop Chauhan
ISBN 1-899066-41-1
Paperback, 220 pages

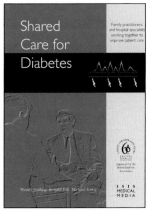

Shared Care for Diabetes
Wendy Gatling, Ronald Hill and Michael Kirby
ISBN 1-899066-25-X
Paperback, 280 pages

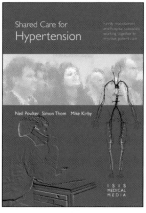

Shared Care for Hypertension
Neil Poulter, Simon Thom and Mike Kirby
ISBN 1-899066-80-2
Paperback, 200 pages

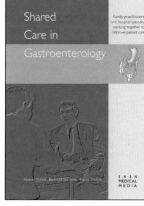

Shared Care in Gastroenterology
Simon Travis, Richard Stevens and Harry Dalton
ISBN 1-899066-40-3
Paperback, 230 pages

ISIS MEDICAL MEDIA Definitive medical publishing for healthcare professionals

The Shared Care Series from ISIS

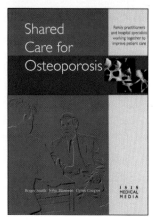

Shared Care for Osteoporosis
Roger Smith, John Harrison and Cyrus Cooper
ISBN 1-899066-26-8
Paperback, 140 pages

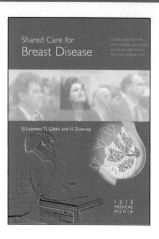

Shared Care for Breast Disease
Samuel Leinster, Trevor Gibbs and Hilary Downey
ISBN 1-901865-57-6
Paperback, 160 pages

ORDER FORM

Please send me (indicate quantity in box on left, and cost on line on right):

Qty	Title	Total (£)
	Shared Care for ENT – *Chris Milford and Aled Rowlands* £22.50/$27.95	
	Shared Care for Prostatic Diseases 2nd Ed – *Roger Kirby, John Fitzpatrick, Michael Kirby and Andrew Fitzpatrick* £22.50/$27.95	
	Shared Care in Gastroenterology – *Simon Travis, Richard Stevens and Henry Dalton* £22.50/$27.95	
	Shared Care for Diabetes – *Wendy Gatling, Ronald Hill and Michael Kirby* £22.50/$27.95	
	Shared Care for Hypertension – *Neil Poulter, Simon Thom and Mike Kirby* £22.50/$27.95	
	Shared Care for Asthma – *Mark Levy, Jon Couriel, Roland Clark, Stephen Holgate and Anoop Chapman* £22.50/$27.95	
	Shared Care for Osteoporosis – *Roger Smith, John Harrison and Cyrus Cooper* £22.50/$27.95	
	Shared Care for Breast Disease – *Samuel Leinster, Trevor Gibbs and Hilary Downey* £22.50/$27.95	
	Books total	
	Postage and packing UK - please add £1.50 per title ordered Rest of the world - please add £3.00/$5.00 per title ordered	
	Total payable	

DELIVER TO:

Name

Inst./Co.

Address

Postcode

Telephone

Fax

E-mail

Visa/Mastercard/American Express

Acct. No. ☐☐☐☐ ☐☐☐☐ ☐☐☐☐ ☐☐☐☐

Exp. Date ☐☐/☐☐

Name of cardholder

Signature

☐ If you need an invoice before payment can be sent, please check here. Book(s) will be sent as soon as payment is received.

ORDERING

Customers outside the US
Isis Medical Media Ltd,
59 St Aldates, Oxford, OX1 1ST
Tel: +44 (0) 1865 202 939   Fax: +44 (0) 1865 202 940
E-mail: info@isismedical.com

Customers in the US
Isis Medical Media,
Books International Inc., P. O. Box 605,
Herndon, VA 20172
Tel: +1 703 661 1500   Fax: +1 703 661 1501
Customer service contact: Beth Prester